Consultant in clinical research
Paris

Alain SPRIET, M.D.Ph.D.

Consultant in clinical research
Paris

Thérèse DUPIN-SPRIET, Pharm.D.

Pharmacologist
Paris

Pierre SIMON, M.D.

Methodology of clinical drug trials

Second, revised edition

Translated by :
Robert COLUZZI, M.D.
John YOUNG, M.D.
Richard EDELSTEIN, M.D.
Michael WEINTRAUB M.D.

With a preface by
Fernand SAUER
Head of "Pharmaceuticals"
Commission of the European Communities

KARGER

Basel - Freiburg - Paris - London - New York - New Delhi - Bangkok - Singapore -Tokyo - Sydney

First English edition, Karger 1985

**Also by Alain Spriet, Thérèse Dupin-Spriet
and Pierre Simon**

Méthodologie des essais cliniques des médicaments
3ème édition, Karger 1993

**Other books by Alain Spriet
and Thérèse Dupin-Spriet**

Good practice of clinical drug trials,
1st edition, Karger 1992

Bonnes pratiques des essais cliniques des médicaments,
1ère édition, Karger 1990

Contents

Preface

The requirements for the demonstration of the quality, safety and efficacy of medicinal products have been considerably upgraded over the last few years in the European Community and are now fully recognised throughout the world. Progress has been particularly important in the field of clinical trials, as compared to the situation prevailing in most Member States before the start of European harmonization.

Pharmacologists and clinical experts, appointed by the national registration authorities, meet regularly within the "efficacy" working party set up by the Committee for Proprietary Medicinal Products. Under the chairmanship of Professor Jean-Michel Alexandre, this working party has systematically codified the principles and methodology of clinical trials in some twenty guidelines for applicants for marketing authorizations, which were published in 1989 and 1990 and are mentionned in the present handbook.

These European guidelines deal with specific therapeutic classes such as anticancer, anti-anginal and antidepressant drugs, topical corticosteroids, etc... They also cover general topics such as clinical trials in children and in the elderly, and good clinical practice from both the ethical and methodological point of view. The guidelines provide for a common implementation and interpretation of the mandatory requirements laid down in the Community directives, mainly Directive 91/507/EEC on norms and protocols for the conduct of analytical, pharmaco-toxicological and clinical tests for medicinal products.

These common requirements are designed to protect public health, to promote the coordination of national marketing authorization procedures and to constitute the foundations of the future system of European authorizations foreseen by the Community Institutions. They also represent the starting point of an ambitious programme for international pharmaceutical harmonization between Europe, the United-States and Japan, which was initiated in 1991 to avoid the unnecessary duplication of drug testing, in particular of clinical trials, for ethical reasons and to reduce the cost of pharmaceutical research worldwide.

This European and international harmonization process is not taking place in isolation. Indeed, a large network of scientists from academia or industry is frequently consulted by the competent regulatory authorities. There is also an obvious need for the results of this process to be made available in a clear and comprehensive didactic form. The authors of the present handbook have already made a significant personal contribution to clinical research and training in France and Europe.

For all these reasons, I am delighted to give a European introduction to the second edition of this volume on methodology for clinical trials with medicinal products, by Alain Spriet, Thérèse Dupin-Spriet and Pierre Simon, which represents a very useful reference handbook for researchers, doctors, industrialists and students, as well as for clinical experts involved in international consultations.

Fernand SAUER

Head of "Pharmaceuticals"
Commission of the European Communities

1- Introduction

This book is intended essentially as a didactic tool for all those who wish to develop, conduct or interpret clinical drug trials.

Every effort has been made to avoid both oversimplification and jargon that might be confusing to the non-specialist. We have drawn attention to the paradoxes and contradictions that exist between the ideal conditions of a clinical trial and the practical constraints, and we have also stressed that common sense should guide the investigator in deciding where to draw the line between a necessary and an unacceptable compromise.

Acceptance of new therapeutic modalities increasingly demands a systematic approach to obtaining *convincing evidence*. All practicing physicians are therefore called upon either to participate in therapeutic trials or to interpret their results. This account of the methods used to systematize the data obtained in a trial and to allow their strict interpretation is therefore intended to provide an understanding all the seemingly unimportant details in which organizers of clinical trials appear to take such delight: they are the price to pay to obtain interpretable results.

The general rules discussed in this book are equally applicable to the study of new treatments and to the re-evaluation of "proven" treatments which, although their *efficacy* may have been demonstrated, may nevertheless require further study concerning their long-term benefits versus their hazards.

1. STAGES IN THE STUDY OF A NEW DRUG

The clinical study of a *new drug* (which must of course be initiated after adequate animal studies have been completed so as to test only the most promising compounds in man), can be divided into several phases such as defined in the following classification:

1.1. Phase 1

• In phase I, the drug is administered to humans for the very first time in order to establish a rough idea of the dose to be administered.
One of the main goals is to detect potentially harmful adverse effects and to determine the doses at which they occur.

These studies require the utmost care, close clinical observation and laboratory monitoring, and the participation of qualified clinical pharmacologists. The initial dose chosen will be very small, based on the data derived from pharmacological, pharmacokinetic and toxicological studies in animals. The choice may also be guided by what is known about similar compounds already in therapeutic use. For example, the initial dose might represent one-hundredth of the dose per kilogram body weight that produces the first detectable effects in the most sensitive animal species tested.

Dose escalation proceeds very slowly; impatience or undue haste may create unnecessary risks for the persons who are subjects in the trial. The next highest dose should only be tested after all the clinical and biological data on the previous dose have been analyzed.

Dose escalation techniques have not yet been strictly codified. The choice depends on the therapeutic class involved. The usual recommendation is to use a geometric progression, with a multiplication factor of 2 (from one to two) sometimes 4, if one wishes to accelerate the process or 1.5 if, on the other hand, one wishes to be more cautious.

An important dose to be determined is the one which produces an effect that is clinically or biologically detectable, whether it is a therapeutic effect or an adverse event.

Single doses should always be tested before repeated doses.

Generally speaking, for this initial phase in which a therapeutic effect is not expected - low doses, single administration - it is preferable to recruit *healthy volunteers* since, should an unexpected and potentially dangerous reaction occur, it is more readily manageable in an individual in good health. Moreover, in this early "escalation" approach to dosage these subjects constitute a relatively reproducible model. In institutions conducting phase 1 trials, adequate facilities for clinical and biological monitoring are mandatory.

In some instances, it is possible to call on sick patients suffering from the disorder for which the new drug is intended. This may be done to the extent that prior withdrawal of previous treatment and administration of very low initial doses (not expected to have a therapeutic effect) are not contra indicated, or if administration of the test drug to healthy volunteers is deemed hazardous (this is the case in particular for antineoplastic agents).

• Phase 1 also includes metabolic and pharmacokinetic studies (with single and then repeated administration) although these studies do not belong exclusively to phase 1 and may be pursued during subsequent phases. In particular, the bioavailability of different pharmaceutical formulations and the identification of metabolites may be studied later. The methodology of phase 1 studies constitutes a highly specialized branch of clinical pharmacology and is beyond the scope of this discussion. These studies are most commonly conducted on healthy volunteers. But it is sometimes very important to conduct such studies in patient populations which may prove to be highly susceptible to them, such as patients with impaired kidney or liver function or in the very elderly.

1.2. Phase 2

During phase 2, the drug's potential therapeutic usefulness is evaluated in rigorously conducted trials by *administering it for limited periods to small numbers* of patients that must be as homogeneous as possible.

1.3. Phase 3

In phase 3, administration of the drug is extended to a *larger and more varied patient population*. Here, attention is turned to the question of the *representativeness of the patients* treated. Also, the duration of administration is increased and may last up to 6 or even 12 months with drugs intended for chronic administration. Finally, comparisons are undertaken with standard proven treatment modalities.

1.4. Phase 4

This phase begins after the new drug has been made commercially available. It may encompass very large-scale studies under usual conditions of use, studies intended to take into account changes in methodology (up-dating of the clinical file) and all studies designed to detect, elucidate and if possible prevent rare and serious adverse effects that may have gone unrecognized in the clinical trials performed previously on smaller numbers of patients and for limited periods of time. Finally, additional more specific studies may be undertaken to investigate or increase knowledge of some pharmacological effects.

Regardless of this, only studies conducted in the country where the new drug has been registered, for the *indication* and *dosage* for which registration approval was granted and with the *pharmaceutical formulation* registered are part of phase 4 trials. Any other program of clinical research on this drug is a return to the preceding phases of the trial.

2. CONTROLLED CLINICAL TRIALS

As a rule, an observed clinical effect cannot be *attributed* to a given treatment unless the observation has been made in a comparative manner with regard to a *control group* or treatment. The trial is then referred to as *confirmatory* (of the hypothesis tested).

This does not mean that uncontrolled or non-comparative trials should not be done, but simply that they do not yield the same sort of information.

The purpose of uncontrolled trials is *exploratory*, or *"hypotheses-generating"*. Such trials are designed to discover or demonstrate something that must be subsequently proved by "controlled" trials. Comparative and non-comparative trials may be appropriate at any stage in the study of a new drug.

2.1. During phase 1

Metabolic and pharmacokinetic studies do not always have to be comparative; on the other hand, trials intended to prove a pharmacodynamic effect should preferably be conducted in comparison with a placebo. In any case, a placebo provides controls for hazards such as environmental or epidemiologic factors: i.e. variations in ambient temperature, a minor viral infection, or unrecognized systematic laboratory errors...

2.2. During phase 2

"Pilot" trials designed to prepare controlled trials by evaluating the feasibility of the proposed protocol may be conducted non-comparatively, with neither control group nor control treatment.

Trials intended to *prove* a therapeutic effect must be comparative, more often with a placebo comparison first and/or comparing several different doses. Such controlled trials providing unquestionable proof of the compound's therapeutic efficacy are, indeed, indispensable before consideration can be given to the following phase.

2.3. During phase 3

Trials designed to compare the short-term or medium-term efficacy of the new treatment with that of one or more standard treatments, must be comparative.

Depending on therapeutic class and indications, extended trials will be conducted in comparison with a placebo or "a standard drug". On the other hand, extended trials lasting several months designed chiefly to detect side effects and in particular relatively common late-onset effects, need not be comparative.

2.4. During phase 4

It is unreasonable to include a control group in very large-scale studies that are intended primarily to detect rare and serious, or unsuspected adverse events as early as possible. If the cause-effect relationship is not obvious for some of these reactions, additional studies may be considered. The methodology of these cohort studies differs somewhat from that of therapeutic trials in the strict sense of the term and will not be dealt with in this book.

On the other hand, most studies designed to update the clinical file must be comparative trials.

Finally, if there is some uncertainty concerning the benefits versus the hazards of prolonged treatment, a large-scale comparative trial lasting several years may be necessary.

3. THE FUNDAMENTALS OF CLINICAL TRIALS METHODOLOGY

At least a working knowledge of a number of fields is necessary to enable one to understand the constraints imposed by the methodology of clinical trials in the choice of persons who are subjects in the trial, the dispensing of treatment, collection of data and analysis of results. The planning of a clinical trial should be *a team effort* with the participation of a clinician, a pharmacologist, a pharmacokineticist, a specialist in pharmaceutical formulations, a statistician, a quality assurance officer, and an ethics committee.

3.1. Clinical data

A sound knowledge of the nosology of the illness treated, its clinical forms, prognostic factors, evaluation techniques and the currently available therapies is indispensable for the accurate definition of patients and the collection of reliable, evaluable and relevant data.

The general principles of therapeutic trials outlined in this work are applicable regardless of the type of disorder studied. They are, nevertheless, insufficient for the understanding of a trial in a specialized field. In this case, it is necessary to consult specialized treatises on the subject when they are available (a list is given at the end of this introduction) and refer to trials in the literature pertaining to the disorder or symptom.

3.2. Pharmacological data

Knowledge of the compound under study and its known or predictable effects (on the basis similar compounds), enables the determination of optimal dosage, prediction of drug interactions, and to a certain extent, the effects in humans.

3.3. Pharmacokinetic data

Pharmacokinetic data are necessary to indicate the route and schedule of drug administration as well as for deciding on the formulation of each of the compounds compared.

3.4. Knowledge of pharmaceutical formulations

Such knowledge enables one to assess the feasibility of pharmaceutical preparations necessary for the trial (elaboration or modification of pre-existing formulations), in particular to make two different treatments indistinguishable.

3.5. Statistical considerations

Statistical considerations are of vital importance *from the outset* when the trial is being designed, and for several reasons:

- to reduce the variability in the measured effects of the treatments administered so as to increase the chances of detecting a difference between them. From this, the willingness to form *homogeneous* groups or subgroups, to administer treatments under *optimal* conditions, and to *collect* data that are sufficiently *sensitive*, *specific*, and *reproducible*.

- to decrease the risk of bias or systematic errors liable to favor one of the treatments to the detriment of the other or others compared. Thus the necessity to form *comparable* groups avoiding a selection process which consciously or unconsciously will favor one of the treatments, and to standardize the conditions under which the treatments are administered and their effects measured.

- to collect data that can be analyzed with the available statistical techniques. *Even the best statistical analysis cannot salvage poor data.* Conversely, organizers of clinical trials must be warned against calling on amateur statisticians who use simple "all-purpose" methods for want of knowledge of more elaborate techniques that are more relevant to the type of trial, the variables studied, the number of measurements, the number of treatments compared, etc.

- to facilitate the interpretation of results, and particularly to avoid the common confusion between a *non-significant difference* and an *"insignificant" or "negligible" difference*, without taking into account the power of the comparison.

3.6. Knowledge of quality assurance

The person responsible for quality assurance must ensure that all phases of each person's work comply with pre-established standards designed to prevent, detect and correct all errors.

3.7. Ethical preoccupations

It is always necessary to obtain the advice of an independent ethics committee since organizers of a clinical trial, no matter how honest their intent, cannot have a clear and impartial view of a trial that they themselves have designed, nor of a treatment that they hope to be adopted.

Ethical questions will be examined in one of the last chapters of this book, their logical place, since the ethical impact of techniques discussed in earlier chapters must be taken into account.

References

N.B.: The references listed at the end of this introduction concern mainly manuals and brochures on clinical trials, particularly as they relate to different fields of medicine.

GENERAL REFERENCES

1 Anonymous. General consideration for the clinical evaluation of drugs. Washington: U.S. Government Printing Office. Food and Drug Administration, 1977.

2 Bulpitt CJ. Randomised controlled clinical trials. Den Haag: Martinus Nijhoff, 1983.

3 Buncher CR, Tsay JY. Statistics in the pharmaceutical industry. New York: Marcel Dekker, 1981.

4 Fleiss J. The design and analysis of clinical experiments. New York: John Wiley and Sons, 1986.

5 Friedman LM, Furberg CD, De Mets DL. Fundamentals of clinical trials. Boston: John Wright, 1981.

6 Glenny H, Nelmes P. Handbook of clinical drug research. Oxford: Blackwell, 1986.

7 Good CS, Clarke C. The principles and practice of clinical trials. Edinburgh: Churchill Livingstone, 1976.

8 Hamilton M. Lectures on the methodology of clinical research. 2nd edition. Edinburgh: Churchill Livingstone, 1974.

9 Harris EL, Fitzerald JD. The principles and practice of clinical trials. Edinburgh: Churchill Livingstone, 1970.

10 Iber FL, Riley WA, Murray P. Conducting clinical trials. New York: Plenum, 1987.

11 Marciano C. Recherche et développement pharmaceutique. Tome 2, Paris: Editions de Santé, 1989.

12 Matoren GM. The clinical research process in the pharmaceutical industry, New York: Marcel Dekker, 1984.

13 Maxwell C. Clinical trial's protocols. Sutton: Stuart Philip, 1969.

14 Meinert CL. Clinical trials. Design, conduct and analysis. New York: Oxford University Press, 1986.

15 Peace KE. Biopharmaceutical statistics for drug development. New York: Marcel Dekker, 1988.

16 Peto R, Pike MC, Armitage P et al. Design and analysis of randomized clinical trials

requiring prolonged observation of each patient. I. Introduction and design. Br J Cancer 1976; *34*: 585-618.

17 Peto R, Pike MC, Armitage P et al. Design and analysis of randomized clinical trials requiring prolonged observation of each patient. II Analysis and examples. Br J Cancer 1977; *35*: 1-39.

18 Pocock SJ. Clinical trials: a practical approach. New York: John Wiley and Sons, 1983.

19 Schwartz D, Flamnant R, Lellouch J. a) L'essai thérapeutique chez l'homme. Paris: Flammarion, 1970. b) Clinical trials. London: Academic Press, 1980.

20 Shapiro SH, Louis TA. Clinical trials: Issues and approaches. New York: Marcel Dekker, 1983.

21 Spilker B. Guide to clinical interpretation of data. New York: Raven Press, 1986.

22 Spilker B. Guide to clinical studies and developing protocols. New York: Raven Press, 1984.

23 Spilker B. Guide to planning and managing multiple clinical studies. New York: Raven Press, 1987.

24 Spilker B, Schoenfelder J. Presentation of clinical data. New York: Raven Press, 1990.

25 Spriet A. Dupin-Spriet Th. a) Bonne pratique des essais cliniques des médicaments. Bâle: Karger, 1990. b) Good practice of clinical drug trials. Basel: Karger, 1992.

26 Spriet A, Simon P. Clinical trials: rules and errors. In: Hindmarch I, Stonier P, eds. Human psychopharmacology: measures and methods, volume 2. New York: John Wiley and Sons, 1989: 251-69.

27 Tygstrup N, Lachin JM, Juhl E. The randomized clinical trial and therapeutic decisions. New York: Marcel Dekker, 1982.

28 Weiner JM. Issues in the desing and evaluation of medical trials. The Hague: Martinus Nijhoff, 1980.

ANTIBIOTICS

29 Anonymous. Guidelines for the clinical investigation of antibacterial drugs. World Health Organization. Regional Office for Europe. Copenhagen, 1986.

30 Anonymous. Policy statement. Division of anti-infection drug products (Draft). Washington: U.S. Government Printing Office. Food and Drug Administration, 1991.

31 Anonymous. The clinical evaluation of antibacterial drugs. British Society for Antimicrobial Chemotherapy. J Antimicrob Chemoth 1989; *23* (suppl. B): 1-41.

32 Gilbert DN, Beam TR Jr, Kunin CM. The path to new FDA guidelines for clinical evaluation of anti-infective drugs. Reviews of Infectious Diseases 1991; *13* (suppl): 890-4.

33 Harkins RD, Albrecht R. Design and analysis of clinical trials for anti-infective drug products. Drug Information Journal 1990; *24*: 213-24.

34 Lunde I. Guidelines of the World Health Organization for clinical trials with antimicrobial agents. Eur J Clin Microbiol Dis 1990; *9*: 548-51.

35 Norrby SR. The Design of clinical trials with antibiotics. Eur J Clin Microbiol Dis 1990; *9*: 523-9.

ONCOLOGY

36 Anonymous. CPMP working party on efficacy of medicinal products. Note for guidance: Evaluation of anticancer medicinal products in man. Brussels: Commission of the European Communities, 1988

37 Anonymous. Guidelines for the clinical evaluation of antineoplastic drugs. Washington: U.S. Government Printing Office. Food and Drug Administration, 1981.

38 Buyse ME, Staquet MJ, Sylvester RJ. Cancer clinical trials; Oxford: Oxford University Press, 1984

39 Geller N. Design of phase I and II trials in cancer. Drug Information Journal 1990, *24*; 341-9.

40 Storer BE. Design and analysis of phase I clinical trials. Biometrics 1989; *45*: 925-37.

41 Writtes R.E. Antineoplastic agents and FDA regulations. Square pegs for round holes? Cancer Treatment Reports 1987; *71*: 795-805.

CARDIOLOGY

42 Anonymous. Clinical testing requirements for drugs used in symptomatic treatment of chronic heart failure. Brussels: European Communities, 1988.

43 Anonymous. Etude clinique des médicaments destinés au traitement des maladies artérielles périphériques chroniques. Journal Officiel des Communautés Européenes 1987; *L 73*: 30-1.

44 Anonymous. Guidelines for the clinical evaluation of anti-anginal drugs. Washington: U.S. Government Printing Office. Food and Drug Administration (Draft), 1989.

45 Anonymous. Guidelines for the clinical evaluation of antiarhythmic drugs. Washington: U.S. Government Printing Office. Food and Drug Administration (Draft), 1989.

46 Anonymous. Guidelines for the clinical investigation of antianginal drugs. Copenhagen: World Health Organization, 1984.

47 Anonymous. Guidelines for the clinical investigation of antihypertensive drugs. Copenhagen: World Health Organization, 1984.

48 Anonymous. Médicaments anti-angineux. Journal Officiel des Communautés Européenes, 1987; *L 73*: 37-40.

49 Anonymous. Proposed guidelines for the clinical evaluation of anti-hypertensive drugs (Draft). Washington: U.S. Government Printing Office. Food and Drug Administration, 1988.

50 Anonymous. Proposed guidelines for the clinical evaluation of congestive heart failure (Draft). Washington: U.S. Government Printing Office. Food and Drug Administration, 1987.

51 Boissel JP, Klimt R. Essais contrôlés multicentres. Principes et problèmes. Paris: INSERM, 1979.

52 McMahon FG. Principle and techniques of human research and therapeutics V. Cardiovascular drugs. Mount Kisco: Futura, 1974.

PHASE I

53 Ingram D. An introduction to human volunteer studies. Richmond: P.J.B. Publication, 1989.

54 Kuemmerle HP, Shibuya TK, Kimura E. Problems of clinical pharmacology in therapeutic research, Phase I. München: Urban-Schwarzenberg, 1977.

55 Metzler CM, Vanderlugt JT. Medical and statistical design issues in clinical pharmacology. Drug Information Journal, 1990; *24*: 281-8.

56 Posvar EL, Sedman A.J. New Drugs: first time in man. J Clin Pharmacol 1989; *29*: 961-6.

PSYCHO-PHARMACOLOGY

57 Anonymous. Clinical investigations of antidepressant drugs. Brussels: European Communities, 1987.

58 Anonymous. Guidelines for the clinical evaluation of antianxiety drugs. Washington: U.S. Government Printing Office. Food and Drug Administration, 1977.

59 Anonymous. Guidelines for the clinical evaluation of antidepressant drugs. Washington: U.S. Government Printing Office. Food and Drug Administration, 1977.

60 Anonymous. Guidelines for the clinical evaluation of psychoactive drugs in infants and children. Washington: U.S. Government Printing Office. Food and Drug Administration, 1979.

61 Anonymous. Guidelines for the clinical investigation of antidepressant drugs. Copenhagen: World Health Organization, 1984.

62 Guelfi JD, Dreyfus JF, Pull CB. Les essais thérapeutiques en psychiatrie: méthodologie, éthique et législation. Masson: Paris, 1978.

63 Hindmarch I, Stonier PD. Human psychopharmacology: measures and method. New York: John Wiley and Sons. Volume 1 (1987), volume 2 (1989), volume 3 (1990).

64 Levine J. Coordinating clinical trials in psychopharmacology. Rockville: N.I.M.H., 1979.

65 Levine J, Schiele BC, Bouthilet L. Principles and problems in establishing the efficacy of psychotropic agents. Washington: Public Health Service. Publication No 2138, 1971.

66 McMahon FG. Principle and techniques of human research and therapeutics VIII. Psychopharmacological agents. Mount Kisco: Futura, 1975.

67 Nicholson PA, Lader MA. Proceedings of a symposium on the evaluation of psychotropic drugs. Br J Clin Pharmacol 1976, 3: 1-108.

68 Raskin A. How to investigate a new antidepressant. In: Diagnosis and treatment of depression. Paris: Medsi McGraw-Hill, 1987.

69 Winterborn JR. Guidelines for clinical trials of psychotropic drugs. Pharmakopsychiatrie, Neuro-psychopharmakologie 1977; 10: 205-31.

RHEUMATOLOGY

70 Anonymous. Guidelines for clinical evaluation of agents used in the treatment or prevention of osteoporosis (Draft). Washington: U.S. Government Printing Office. Food and Drug Administration, 1985.

71 Anonymous. Guidelines for the clinical evaluation of anti-inflammatory drugs (adults and children). US Department of Health and Human Services. Washington: US Government Printing Office. Food and Drug Administration, 1988 (reviewed).

72 Anonymous. Médicaments anti-inflammatoires non-stéroïdiens pour le traitement des maladies chroniques. Journal Officiel des Communautés Européenes 1987; L 73: 22-3.

73 Dumonde DC, Jasani MK. Recognition of anti-rheumatic drugs. Lancaster: MTP Press, 1978.

74 Klippel JH, Decker JL. Clinical trials in the rheumatic diseases. Clinics in Rheumatic Diseases 1983; 9: 489-695.

75 Méry C. L'essai thérapeutique des anti-inflammatoires en rhumatologie. Paris: Laboratoires Dausse, 1978.

MISCELLANEA

76 Anonymous. Clinical investigation of medicinal products in children. Journal Officiel des Communautés Européenes 1988; L 73: 19-21.

77 Anonymous. Clinical investigation of medicinal products in the elderly. Brussels: European Communities, 1987.

78 Anonymous. Corticoïdes à usage cutané. Journal Officiel des Communautés Européenes 1987; L 73: 41-6.

79 Anonymous. Draft guideline for the design of clinical trials for evaluation of safety and efficacy of allergenic products for therapeutic use. Washington: US Government Printing Office. Food and Drug Administration (Draft), 1988.

80 Anonymous. Examen clinique des contraceptifs oraux. Journal Officiel des Communautés Européenes 1987; L 73: 10-5.

81 Anonymous. Exigences en matière d'essais cliniques de médicaments pour utilisation à long terme. Journal Officiel des Communautés Européenes 1988; L 73: 19-21.

82 Anonymous. Guidelines for the clinical evaluation of antiacid drugs. Washington: US Government Printing Office. Food and Drug Administration, 1977.

83 Anonymous. Guidelines for the clinical evaluation of anticonvulsant drugs. Washington: US Government Printing Office. Food and Drug Administration, 1977.

84 Anonymous. Guidelines for the clinical evaluation of antidiarrhea drugs. US. Washington: US Government Printing Office. Food and Drug Administration, 1977.

85 Anonymous. Guidelines for the clinical evaluation of bronchodilatation drugs. Washington: US Government Printing Office. Food and Drug Administration, 1978.

86 Anonymous. Guidelines for the clinical evaluation of drugs in infants and children. Washington: US Government Printing Office. Food and Drug Administration, 1977.

87 Anonymous. Guidelines for the clinical evaluation of drugs to prevent, control and/or treat periodontal disease. Washington: US Government Printing Office. Food and Drug Administration, 1978.

88 Anonymous. Guidelines for the clinical evaluation of drugs to prevent dental caries. Washington: US Government Printing Office. Food and Drug Administration, 1978.

89 Anonymous. Guidelines for the clinical evaluation of gastric secretory depressant drugs. Washington: US Government Printing Office. Food and Drug Administration, 1977.

90 Anonymous. Guidelines for the clinical evaluation of general anesthetics. Washington: US Government Printing Office. Food and Drug Administration, 1977.

91 Anonymous. Guidelines for the clinical evaluation of GI motility modifying drugs. Washington: US Government Printing Office. Food and Drug Administration, 1978.

92 Anonymous. Guidelines for the clinical evaluation of hypnotic drugs. Washington: US Government Printing Office. Food and Drug Administration, 1977.

93 Anonymous. Guidelines for the clinical evaluation of laxative drugs. Washington: US Government Printing Office. Food and Drug Administration, 1978.

94 Anonymous. Guidelines for the clinical evaluation of lipid-altering agents in adults and children. Washington: US Government Printing Office. Food and Drug Administration, 1980.

95 Anonymous. Guidelines for the clinical evaluation of general anesthetics. Washington: US Government Printing Office. Food and Drug Administration, 1977.

96 Anonymous. Guidelines for the clinical evaluation of radiopharmaceutical drugs. Washington: US Government Printing Office. Food and Drug Administration, 1977.

97 Anonymous. Guidelines for the clinical investigation of antiepileptic drugs. Copenhagen: World Health Organization, 1985.

98 Anonymous. Guidelines for the format and content of the clinical and statistical sections of new drug applications. Washington: US Government Printing Office. Food and Drug Administration, 1988.

99 Anonymous. Guideline for the study of drugs likely to be used in the elderly. Washington: US Government Printing Office. Food and Drug Administration, 1989.

100 Anonymous. Produits anti-épileptiques/anti-convulsivants. Journal Officiel des Communautés Européenes 1987; L 73: 24-6.

101 Anonymous. Recommendations de base pour la conduite d'essais cliniques de médicaments pour la Communauté Européene. Bruxelles: Communautés Européenes, 1987.

102 Anonymous. The clinical investigation of drugs for the long-term prophylactic management of asthma. Copenhagen: World Health Organization, 1988.

103 McMahon F.G. Principle and techniques of human research and therapeutics IX. Evlauation of gastro-intestinal, pulmonary, anti-inflammatory and immunological agents. Mount Kisco: Futura, 1975.

104 McMahon F.G. Principle and techniques of human research and therapeutics VI. Endocrino-metabolic drugs. Mount Kisco: Futura, 1974.

105 Méry C. L'essai thérapeutique des antalgiques. Paris: Diamant, 1981.

106 Nicholson PA, Prescott LF, Coulston F. Proceedings of a symposium on mild analgesics. Br J Clin Pharmacol 1980; 10: suppl. 2, 209 S - 412 S.

2 - Principles of the controlled trial

SUMMARY

Evidence for the efficacy of a drug can be obtained through a "controlled" trial involving groups of comparable patients studied simultaneously. Variations between subjects may suffice to account for differences observed between groups (sampling errors) and such variations must be taken into account when interpreting the results.

In addition to statistical "errors" (false differences or alternately, concealed differences), systematic errors or bias favoring one treatment to the detriment of another may distort the comparison.

Before undertaking a trial, a single, clear and "explicit question" must be formulated.

A difference can only be proven (with an acceptable risk of error) by rejecting a working "null" hypothesis of no difference. If the difference is substantial compared to the variability of the responses, the probability that this difference is due to sampling error is low. Such a difference is said to be statistically significant and the null hypothesis can be rejected.

On the opposite case, all that can be said is that there is no evidence for any difference (unless if, by using the appropriate calculation, it can be proven that any possible difference cannot be large).

The results of a trial can only be generalized to similar patients receiving the same treatments under similar conditions. A trial can only answer the question it was designed for.

Finally, non-reproducible results may be due to bias, statistical "errors" or differences in the quality of similar trials.

Before a drug can be made available for wide-scale use, its effects must be carefully evaluated in patients with the illness for which the drug will eventually be prescribed. Experience has shown that these effects are never exactly alike in all individuals and all circumstances. It is necessary therefore, to reason in terms of groups of patients rather than in terms of individuals.

The benefits of the drug must also be weighed against alternative forms of treatment or no treatment at all: this implies that the drug be *compared* to one or more treatments in *comparable subjects* and under *comparable circumstances.*

Should a difference in efficacy or adverse effects emerge from such a comparison, it must be interpreted carefully. Is the difference observed due to external factors totally unrelated to the treatment? Has chance favored one of the treatments evaluated? It must be conceded that these are questions that cannot be answered with absolute certainty and one is therefore led to take account of possible errors and their probability. In other words, one must reason in *statistical terms.* This can only be done properly if there are not too many questions to be answered in the course of a trial. One should not, therefore, be overambitious, and it is wise to attempt to answer *only one question* per trial (and to consider designing other trials for other questions).

Putting aside ethical questions for the moment, here then, in a nutshell, is the overall view of a *controlled trial* (so-called because it involves comparison with a "control" group or "control" treatment): formulation a priori of a single, explicit question, reasoning in terms of groups rather than individuals, comparison, statistical analysis and conclusions (carefully drawn because of the relative uncertainty).

The words "control" and "controlled" are ambiguous. In the field of clinical research alone, Feinstein (6) has identified 12 different meanings including: balanced or compensated (as in controlled diabetes); verification (as in quality control); stabilization before a test or an investigation (baseline, control period); comparative (control group or control treatment).

In the term "controlled trial" it is this latter meaning that is intended, although it may also be considered that if the required degree of stringency in the design and performance of the trial has been observed, "controllable" sources of error have been eliminated. The term a "well controlled trial" can be understood in this light.

The technical aspects of the problem (formation of groups, description of methods, standardization of assessment criteria, design of the trial, collection and analysis of data) which will be detailed in writing in a protocol, derive from these principles and it is appropriate to present these in greater detail.

1. WHY CONDUCT CONTROLLED TRIALS?

One may well ask why require so much rigor in clinical trials when it has long been shown that gradually acquired experience combined with a certain insight can achieve the same result? Insulin and penicillin were discovered long before the era of controlled trials and no-one questions their efficacy.

On the other hand, other older treatments continue to be used without proof of efficacy and without convincing evidence.

More important, treatments once unanimously believed to be effective were subsequently proven to be of no use, or at least of dubious efficacy after being submitted to a controlled trial. Should estrogens still be prescribed indiscriminately in the treatment of prostate cancer patients with a high cardiac risk, despite the results of the Veterans Administration trials (1)?

Conversely, treatments that were previously the object of debate have proven to be remarkably useful in the light of controlled trials. One such example is the treatment of hypertension, which has come to be considered as indispensable following the demonstration that treatment markedly reduced mortality (2)

Last and most important, while it is true that *revolutionary* advances in therapeutics may not require stringent testing to prove their worth, it must be humbly recognized that such advances are very rare occurrences, indeed. In the vast majority of cases, therapeutic progress comes about as a result of the accumulation of minor improvements that require careful observation and consequently, strict methodology (15). Even in the case of a new compound claimed to be prodigiously effective, it is generally difficult to ascertain the optimal administration modalities, the optimal dosage schedule, and the indications of greatest, little or no interest, without the precise data derived from carefully conducted trials.

2. WHY REASON IN TERMS OF GROUPS?

The clinician often feels that since each patient is unique, general conclusions valid for all patients cannot be drawn from a group in which the fate of each individual is disregarded. Unquestionably, there is some truth in all of this; each patient is different, general rules are not necessarily applicable to all patients and the results of treatment in an individual patient cannot be disregarded.

However, for want of infallible general rules, it is essential to have some idea of what can be accomplished *on the average* with various treatments so as to give preference to the one that can reasonably be expected to have the greatest chance of being effective in a given situation.

This will not eliminate the clinician's need, in many cases, for trying several treatments before finding the one that is most suitable for an individual patient, but at least he does not have to set out totally in the dark.

If controlled trials have been performed, they provide the physician with systematically collected data which, although *specific for the population studied*, nonetheless are generalizable to some degree.

It is precisely because patients are individuals, each one different in his own right, that a treatment must be assessed in terms of *probable results*, i.e. by statistical reasoning derived from study of a group.

3. WHAT TO COMPARE WITH WHAT?

The usefulness of a treatment cannot be appraised in the absolute sense but only in *relative* terms, i.e. by comparison. One possibility might be to treat a group of patients with a new drug and to compare the results with those observed in patients formerly treated by another drug. This is referred to as a "historical" comparison (historical meaning at a previous time).

Unfortunately, this approach generally carries a high risk of distorting the results. Recruitment of patients may have changed (patients referred to an institution may have a better or worse prognosis than previously), diagnostic criteria may have evolved or become more refined, those responsible for patient care may have acquired greater experience in screening for or classifying the illness, or in evaluating its prognosis. Usually prescribed concomitant treatments may have changed; finally, the illness itself may be subject to seasonal or secular trends.

For all these reasons, *simultaneous comparison* is generally preferred which implies *studying comparable groups* of patients at the same time. To ensure that the *groups* are strictly comparable, it would be ideal to have strictly comparable *subjects*: the unique nature of each individual makes this condition an unachievable utopia.

The use of groups formed post hoc based on large computerized medical data bases is sometimes specified to compare treatments. This method is useful for generating hypotheses. It cannot test them because of the risk of systematic errors related to the choice of treatments, changes in prescriptions over time and to methods of evaluation and to the non-homogeneous origin of non-standardized data (6).

4. DIFFERENCES BETWEEN INDIVIDUALS AND BETWEEN GROUPS

Patients differ from each other not only in their initial pretreatment status but also in their response to treatment. The greater the difference between the individuals in a group, the more variable the anticipated difference between responses to therapy. Consequently, the more difficult it will be to draw general conclusions from the results observed in the group.

To evaluate the results of a treatment, it is therefore desirable to choose relatively homogeneous groups in which there is as little variability as possible.

While many factors affecting the outcome of a trial are unknown, certain patient characteristics can reasonably be considered as a source of this variability. It is therefore important to list these factors so that they can be taken into account either for interpreting individual responses or for reducing the lack of homogeneity among subjects and results.

Table I

Sources of variability

1. Characteristics of the disorder treated:
- nosology (unambiguous definition of the illness)
- clinical forms (according to symptoms, course, etiology)
- prior treatments and results

2. Associated illnesses and treatments thereof

3. Demographic and physiologic characteristics of the subjects:
age, sex, weight, height, ethnic background, psychological profile, socio-economic status, diet, physical exercise, etc.

4. External factors:
medical staff, climate, season, environment, inpatient or outpatient status, occupation.

5. Treatment:
dosage, route of administration, schedule, compliance with therapy, drug formulation, bioavailability.

The list presented in table I is not exhaustive and the factors contained in it are not relevant in all cases; nonetheless, it gives an idea of *the questions that should be asked in order to interpret the variability of results.*

Schematically, different influences may be represented as the sum of the factors (Table II) whose cancelling out makes it possible to estimate the difference between the treatments compared. This cancelling out effect is achieved partly:

- by standardization (similar recruitment in both study groups, treatment administered under the same conditions, the same assessment criterion...),

- and partly by an adequate number of subjects. Indeed, the higher the number of subjects involved, the greater the probability that variations in the opposite direction will be cancelled out (provided that treatments are randomly assigned to patients, a provision which will be discussed in chapter 5).

Table II

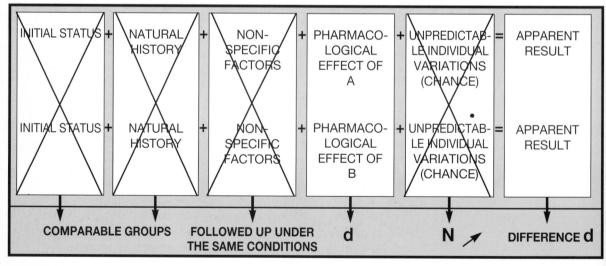

A very important consequence of the lack of homogeneity among subjects in a group is that *variations between individuals may lead to variations between groups.* These variations are then referred to as *sampling errors* and depend on the selection of subjects who make up the patient "sample", since all existing (or future) patients cannot be included in the trial.

Statistical reasoning consists in comparing the differences between groups to variations in individuals within groups. If there is a small difference between groups with respect to individual variability, the latter may be sufficient to explain this difference. On the other hand, if there is a large difference, minor variability is not enough to explain the difference.

Finally, individual variations in opposite directions tend to cancel each other out at the group level, this being greatest in large groups. This fact serves to emphasize the importance of therapeutic trials carried out on large numbers of subjects.

5. ASKING THE RIGHT QUESTION (DEFINING THE AIM OF THE TRIAL)

It is not possible, in the *same* trial, to compare a new treatment to a "control treatment", study its effects separately on isolated symptoms, define dosage and optimal duration of therapy, identify the preferred indications, study drug interactions to be recommended or avoided, define precautions for use in all categories of subjects (according to age, renal function, etc.). A *single precise question* must be defined around which the trial will be built (selection of subjects, method of administration, data collected, etc.).

Indeed, the greater the number of questions asked, the greater the chance of errors (false differences). More serious still is the fact that probability calculations will be distorted and the degree of error impossible to assess, if multiple, non-independent questions are asked. This does not exclude the possibility of asking subsidiary questions, e.g. on patient tolerability, acceptability, or feasibility, but in this case, the conclusions will not be as "solid".

To avoid cheating in following the single question asked, the objective of the trial must be clearly defined *a priori* in the protocol, before examining the first results (otherwise there may be more or less conscious selection among a number of questions that were not all excluded a priori, but some of which will be eliminated *a posteriori*).

The question asked must be *simple* so that the answer will be *clear* and readily interpretable.

Finally, the question must be *realistic* and compatible with patient recruitment and with the human and material ressources available.

This requires discussion among those involved in the trial (sponsor, organizer, clinician, statistician) *before the work begins*. Such a discussion may conclude that the trial project is not feasible or that the objective must be limited and made less ambitious. It may also lead to the conclusion that the question is too trivial to make the necessary effort worthwhile!

6. INITIAL STATISTICAL REASONING: REJECTING HYPOTHESES

If we wish to show that there is a difference between two treatments, we try to reject the "null" hypothesis i.e. that there is no difference between them. If the results of the trial are incompatible with the hypothesis, it is rejected and the difference between the treatments will be considered too great to be accounted for by sampling error alone, the latter being evaluated by examining differences between the subjects.

An appropriate "statistical test" is then applied *to calculate the chances of this difference being observed if the treatments were strictly equivalent*. In other words, *"what would be the probability of this difference being due to sampling error if the null hypothesis were correct"?*

This test is a calculated dimension:
- proportional to the difference observed (d)
- inversely proportional to variability (V: variance or the square of the standard deviation)
- proportional to the number of subjects (N) which cancels out the influence of the variance on the differences.
This value (a function of d, V, N) is inversely proportional to the probability that the difference is explained by the variance. This probability can itself be calculated using the test value obtained.

If this probability is small (e.g. less than 5 in 100), the difference observed is said to be *statistically significant*. Since probability p is conventionally expressed by a value between 0 (an impossible event) and 1 (a certain event) this is written as $p \leq 0.05$. By convention, it is generally conceded that the probability of error is negliglible when the p value is below this threshold.

The arbitrary nature of this limit (7) will not escape the reader.

$p > 0.05$: not significant
$p \leq 0.05$: significant.

6.1. A "significant" difference is observed

• This does not necessarily mean that the difference is of practical importance. If the conditions are favorable (little variation between a large number of subjects), a minor difference may be demonstrated but only *clinical* judgment can decide whether such a difference is truly meaningful in a medical or therapeutic sense or not. Statistical calculations can be of no help whatsoever in making such a decision.

• The fact that a difference is statistically significant does not mean that it is truly due to a difference in efficacy between the treatments. Although the probability of such a difference being due to sampling error is small, it always exists.

When this occurs, i.e. when an effect is erroneously attributed to a drug, the error committed is called a "type I error" for which a probability α (commonly $\alpha = 0.05$, i.e. 5%) is accepted *a priori by* choosing this threshold as the limit of "significance". Nonetheless, it is always possible to choose another "threshold" of significance (e.g. $\alpha = 0.01$). But the more this threshold is decreased, which makes results more convincing, the higher the number of subjects needed to demonstrate a given difference. A compromise is necessary: $\alpha = 0.05$ is commonly accepted.

• In addition to these two factors (real differences and random fluctuations), there is also the problem of bias: systematic errors which *distort the comparison* by favoring or disfavoring one of the compared treatments. If such a bias comes to the attention of the investigator, one must admit that the results cannot be interpreted. If, however, the results are analyzed (the bias is not apparent) or if a bias has been overlooked, the *conclusions* drawn from the trial *may be false.*

Two meanings of "bias" are often confused:
- a systematic trend influencing recruitment of subjects and limiting the *representativity* of the group studied. This is an inevitable occurrence in a therapeutic trial because only a "random sampling" (in practice impossible to do in this context) makes it possible to form a representative "sample" from "a given population". It should be noted that it is by convention, and improperly so, that groups of subjects enrolled in a controlled trial are referred to as "samples";
- conditions favoring one of the compared therapies: e.g. an unfair dose or time schedule, or data collection favoring observation of favorable results with one of the treatments.

Strictly speaking, initial non-comparability of groups despite randomization is not a bias but a random error. It is important nevertheless, to look for it and to take it in consideration when interpreting results (5,14).

Elimination of bias is one of the reasons for standardization of all phases of the trial.

6.2. If the difference observed is "not significant"

this does not justify the conclusion that the treatments are equivalent since other possibilities exist:

• There may be a real difference concealed by chance sampling: a "type II error".

• The comparison may not be sensitive enough owing to an insufficient number of patients or unfavorable study conditions (dosage too low, assessment criteria insufficiently sensitive, poorly chosen indications, etc.).

An overall view of possible conclusions is shown in table III.

Table III
Interpreting differences between treatments

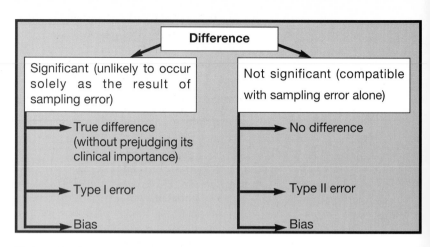

7. SECOND TYPE OF STATISTICAL REASONING: REJECTION OF THE ALTERNATIVE HYPOTHESIS

If the aim is to prove that two treatments are equivalent under the prevailing experimental conditions (e.g. if a new drug is being compared to a previously proven drug), it is necessary to first verify that the null hypothesis has not been rejected.

Furthermore, it must be possible to reject an alternative hypothesis, according to which the difference is equal to Δ. Its value is a compromise between meaningful differences (which one wishes to demonstrate), and negligible differences (that one accepts to ignore). This can be expressed in different fashions: for example "10% more favorable results than with the control treatment", or "a 50% improvement over the result obtained with a placebo".

Two opposite errors can be made in choosing Δ :
- choosing a Δ that is too small and so difficult to detect and requiring an enormous trial to obtain a modest gain;
- choosing a Δ that is too large and thus utopic for a new treatment. Miracles are easy to see but rarely occur!

For this reason, if a prior consensus on a value for Δ is not available, one will have to be obtained before the trial is started.

As it is not possible to prove that two treatments are strictly equal, it can be accepted that they are approximately equivalent if the difference between them does not reach Δ.

The choice of Δ is difficult: indeed any improvement, albeit minor, in the therapeutic result is useful. Unfortunately, the smaller the difference, the harder it is to demonstrate because sampling errors (due to chance alone) can by themselves often be the cause.

In addition, it is necessary to reason in terms of probability: "what are the chances of not observing a significant difference if the real difference between treatments is equal to Δ? Or what is the probability that sampling errors have concealed the difference between treatments if the alternative hypothesis is true?"

Δ is then the difference that one wishes to detect with reasonable chances (e.g. 95%).

Thus, a maximum probability of 5% for β is accepted for a type II error (missing a real difference).

The sensitivity of the comparison depends on the number of subjects in each group: for a given difference Δ, the greater the number of subjects, the smaller becomes the risk of missing the difference.

Furthermore, it is a good idea to calculate *a posteriori* the "power" of the test (probability of observing a significant difference if there really is a difference Δ). It then is often noted that this probability is low and that the absence of statistical significance may well be accounted for by sampling error (type II error).

It is possible to control this risk of error *a priori* by calculating the number of subjects required in each group so that if the true difference is Δ, there is a high degree of probability (1 - β) of detecting it significantly ($p < \alpha$).

β = 0.10 is commonly chosen (i.e. a 10% chance of missing Δ and a 90% chance of detecting it), or even β = 0.20. It then is common to accept to ignore a difference with a higher probability than that of detecting an artifact if α = 0.05. The reason for these choices, which are partly arbitrary, is that in many disorders it is more acceptable to miss the efficacy of "another drug" (there already are several of them) than to suggest the use of an ineffective treatment. In certain illnesses, the converse reasoning may apply. This must be taken into account when choosing α and β.

All possible combinations are summarized in table IV.

Table IV

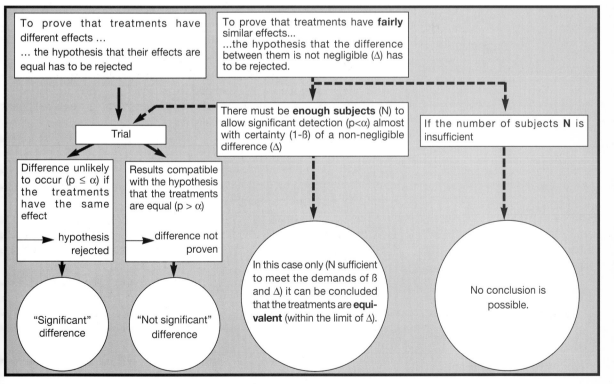

8. ONE-TAILED TEST

Comparisons between treatments can be made more sensitive by a one-tailed test. In this case, one must be certain that one of the treatments can be better than or equal to the other but is certainly not worse. This test offers the advantage of being significant for a given difference using fewer subjects. In practice, this test should be reserved for two cases:
- some comparisons versus placebo (N.B. there are "treatments" that are less effective than placebo),
- a test between two doses of the same product if one is certain of the direction of the possible difference.

Selection of a one-tailed analysis may often be debatable (3, 8, 9, 10, 13) and as a precaution some authors systematically refrain from using it. In case of doubt, a two-tailed test is acceptable even though the protocol called for a one-tailed test. The opposite case is often much more questionable since, in light of the results, it could be possible to artificially convert a non-significant test into a significant one.

9. CONFIDENCE INTERVAL

Another way of analyzing results consists in calculating a zone of uncertainty around a difference observed, in which the true difference should be found.

The amplitude of this zone is:
- proportional to the variability V of results
- inversely proportional to the number of cases N
- inversely proportional to the degree of uncertainty that is accepted (e.g. 5% for a 95% confidence interval).

Generally, this procedure supplements the test (figures 1 and 2):
- prior to the trial, α, β and Δ are set ($\pm\Delta$ for a two-tailed comparison)
- during the trial, data on N' subjects are collected (if possible N' is close to N)
- after the trial:
• the test makes it possible to know whether there is a real difference (significant),
• the confidence interval compares this difference both to H_0, the null hypothesis and to H_1, the alternative hypothesis. It enables to confirm that the difference is real if the interval does not reach zero and that any difference is small if the interval entirely lies between $+\Delta$ and $-\Delta$. Finally if it only reaches one of the boundaries ($+\Delta$ or $-\Delta$), it enables exclusion of a major difference and in the opposite direction to the one observed.

10. GENERALIZATION OF RESULTS

When a trial is undertaken, the aim is to draw conclusions that can be extended to other subjects. Yet, each patient is unique and no trial will ever be able to predict infallibly the outcome in a given patient, of the treatment prescribed.

Results could be theoretically generalized only within a specific population from which the subjects in a trial have been randomly selected. This is impossible in practice. A compromise thus is necessary by analogy. It is acceptable to generalize:
- to subjects with characteristics similar to those in the trial
- cared for under comparable conditions (dosage, duration of treatment, external conditions, activity, diet, etc..).
The value of results obtained in one country for patients in other countries is often questioned. In practice, results differ rarely from one country to another, but the interpretation must take into account:
- differences in dosage due to differences in patient height and weight,
- the influence of climatic and seasonal conditions on the disorder,
- possible genotypic metabolic differences or interference due to dietary or therapeutic habits.

Figure 1

On the horizontal lines individual favorable results (upwards) or unfavorable results (downwards) for two treatments A and B are depicted, schematized by small horizontal lines.

A difference is detected all the more readily:
- if it is large,
- if the variability is smaller,
- if the number of cases is larger,
- if the acceptable probability of a type I error is larger (N.B.: if the difference is detected more often it is also less convincing),
- if the acceptable probability of a type II error is smaller.

The dotted horizontal lines symbolize extreme cases, poorly distributed by chance, which cause the result to "tilt".

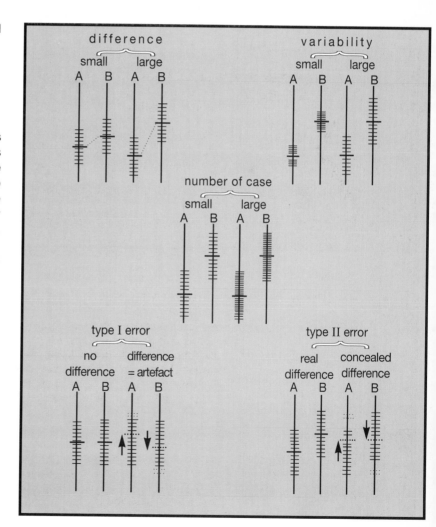

23

Figure 2 Summary of the stages of comparison

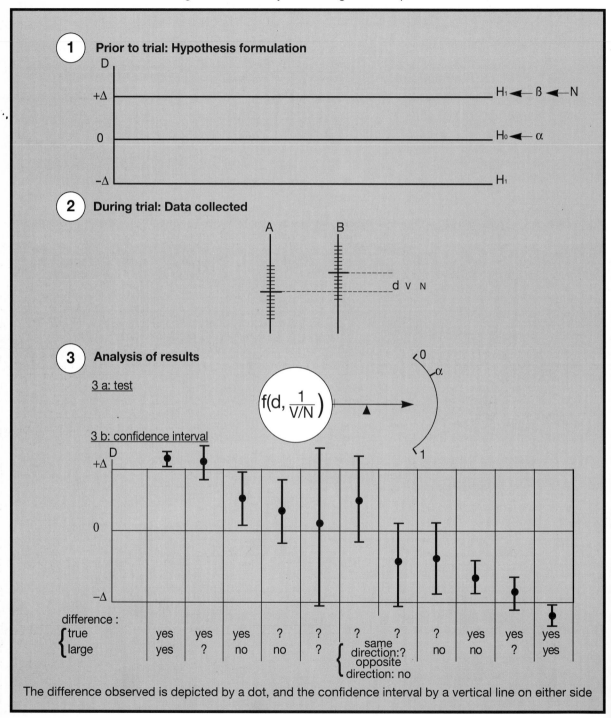

The difference observed is depicted by a dot, and the confidence interval by a vertical line on either side

11. "UNFORESEEN" OBSERVATIONS

If a hypothesis is to be submitted to a valid statistical comparison, it must be formulated *a priori*. A trial thus can only answer *the question for which it was designed*. This does not mean that other findings should be disregarded but strictly speaking, a hypothesis cannot be formulated from unexpected observations and tested statistically by these *same results* (circular reasoning). These then are not confirmatory but rather exploratory results. They require independent confirmation, possibly by a new trial if the question is important (cf table V).

Table V

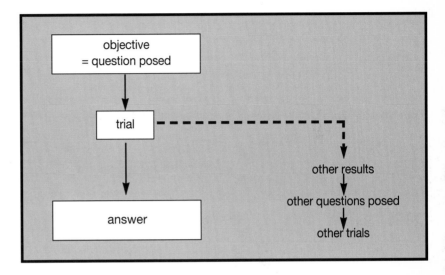

12. ROLE OF NON-CONTROLLED TRIALS

A non-controlled trial cannot demonstrate efficacy since the results can be influenced by: the spontaneous course of the disorder (an improvement or a deterioration), the amount of subjectivity in the most "objective" measurements of efficacy (measurement unconsciously favorable to the preferred hypothesis) and the non-specific effects of treatment (placebo effect or "therapist" effect of the physician).

Nonetheless, non-comparative trials can or should be undertaken in the following circumstances:

- sometimes the very first investigations of toxicity in man designed to establish the safety of the doses that will be used subsequently;

- some "exploratory" trials intended to document effects that will lead to formulating hypotheses or pilot studies of *feasibility*;

- some *purely pharmacokinetic* and metabolic studies whose sole purpose is to determine levels of a drug in biological fluids (if *clinical information* is expected from such studies, inclusion of a control group is preferable);

- long-term toxicity studies, and large-scale studies conducted under "naturalistic" conditions, in particular cohort studies designed to detect serious uncommon adverse effects;

- clinical trials involving *illnesses that are always rapidly fatal* (with little or no exceptions), with no known treatment and in which the aim is to test a potentially curative treatment.

13. REPRODUCIBILITY OF TRIAL RESULTS

It is by no means uncommon for the results of a therapeutic trial to be contradicted by subsequent trials. There may be several reasons for this which are not mutually exclusive:

- a trial may have been conducted in accordance with an inadequately designed protocol that was too vague in its definition of important details (on patient selection criteria, treatment modalities or data collection);

- one of the trials may have been affected by an unrecognized bias;

- sampling errors may have been responsible for the conflicting conclusions even if an identical protocol was complied with and in which there was no bias (risk α of type I error);

- the sample sizes (number of patients) must be taken into consideration because a non-significant difference with few subjects can become significant when the same study is performed with a larger number of patients (risk β or type II error);

- "negative" results - a term often applied to results that do not show a significant difference between two treatments - are less often published (since they are not as readily accepted by journals) than studies that show differences (4);

- finally, in the process for selection of new drug entities there is a tendency to retain those compounds that *initially* produced the most promising results. Among these, some initially promising results may be due to chance alone while other drugs may be rejected for seemingly poor results that also may be the result of chance. This is why the results of subsequent studies are frequently less brilliant that those of early studies, whence the old saying *"when a new drug becomes available hasten to use it while it still works"*.

References

1 Anonymous. Veterans Administration cooperative urological research group. Treatment and survival of patients with cancer of the prostate. Surg Gynec Obstet 1967; *124*: 1011-7.

2 Anonymous. Veterans Administration cooperative study group on antihypertensive agents. Effects of treatment on morbidity in hypertension II Results in patients with diastolic blood pressure averaging 90 through 114 mm Hg. JAMA 1970; *213*: 1143-52.

3 Boissel JP. Some thoughts on two-tailed tests (and two-sided designs). Controlled Clinical Trials 1988; *9*: 385-6.

4 Byar PB. Problems with using observational databases to compare treatments. Statistics in Medicine 1991; *10*: 663-70.

5 Chalmers TC. The control of bias in clinical trials. In: Shapiro SH, Louis TA, eds. Clinical trials issues and approaches. New York: Marcel Dekker, 1983: 115-27.

6 Feinstein AR. Clinical biostatistics XIX. Ambiguity and abuse in the twelve different concepts of "control". Clin Pharmacol Ther 1973; *14*: 112-22.

7 Feinstein AR. Clinical biostatistics. Saint Louis: CV Mosby Company, 1977.

8 Fleiss JL. Some thoughts on two-tailed tests. Controlled Clinical Trials 1987; *8*: 394.

9 Fleiss JL. One-tailed versus two-tailed tests: rebuttal. Controlled Clinical Trials 1988; *10*: 227-30.

10 Goodman S. One-tailed or two-tailed p values? Controlled Clinical Trials 1988; *9*: 387-8.

11 Maxwell C. Clinical trials, reviews, and the journal of negative results. Br J Clin Pharmac 1981; *11*: 15-8.

12 Modell W. On the significance of significant. Clin Pharmacol Ther 1981; *30*: 1-2.

13 Peace KE. Some thoughts on one-tailed tests. Controlled Clinical Trials 1988; *9*: 383-4.

14 Rose G. Bias. Br J Clin Pharmac 1982; *13*: 157-62.

15 Schwartz D. Les essais thérapeutiques. Principes nouveaux et nouvelles orientations. Psychologie médicale 1973; *5*: 651-2.

3 - Selection of subjects

SUMMARY

The requirements and considerations which must be taken into account when selecting subjects for controlled clinical trials include:

• the characteristics of the disease from which the patients suffer should be such that the response to the treatments compared can demonstrate a difference between these treatments if a true difference exists;

• the groups of patients must be sufficiently uniform with regard to the natural history of the disease and its response to treatment (this limits recruitment);

• the groups must, as much as possible, consist of patients who are "representative" of the illness studied (this broadens the recruitment). Since the two requirements of uniformity and representativeness are contradictory, a compromise must be found in agreement with the aims of the study;

• expected patient accrual should be assessed realistically, since it is generally overestimated when the trial is designed;

• ethical principles must be observed if the trial represents a risk for certain categories of patients.

These criteria so defined should be stated in the trial protocol under the headings "eligibility criteria" (definition of the disease studied) and "exclusion criteria" (categories of patients not to be included) and should be formulated so as to be unambiguously reproducible.

Once the objective of the trial has been explicitly defined (and the working hypotheses clearly formulated), the next step is to decide on the type of patients to be included in the trial.

This choice must take into account *several, sometimes contradictory requirements.*

• groups of subjects must be recruited so as to enable differences between treatments to be demonstrated, if they exist (selection adapted to the trial objective);

- the groups must be sufficiently uniform regarding the characteristics relevant to the disorder and the treatments under study. This is important in order to reduce the variability of the responses which in turn makes statistical comparison more sensitive and reduces the possibility of errors;

- to obtain results which, within reasonable limits, can be generalized;

- to define realistic criteria for patient recruitment;

- ethical principles must be adhered to.

1. OPTIMIZING THE CHANCES OF SHOWING A DIFFERENCE

This requirement, the objective of the trial, specifies that an operational definition of the disorder under study and its clinical forms be given.

A definition is operational when it enables unambiguous and reproducible selection (quantified if possible) based on readily identifiable symptoms in the patients. In particular, it is necessary to be precise with regard to the fate of "marginal" or "borderline" cases (16). In addition, this definition must exclude forms of the disorder which are too benign (the potential difference in therapeutic efficacy is small), or too serious (often resistant to all treatments).

Repeated participation of the same subjects in successive trials involving chronic disorders raises two specific problems:

- *the patients may be serious sufferers* who have not responded to several proven treatments: in this case, the chances of success of any other treatment, albeit a novel one, are slim;

- *the patients may be "symptomatic volunteers"*, intermediate between healthy subjects and more seriously ill patients. Their participation has been suggested in psychiatric trials (9) but there is a risk that they may not be representative of "real" patients. They may, however, constitute a convenient model for rapid assessment of new drugs.

Finally, the question of *healthy volunteers* often arises. Certainly there may be legal and ethical problems associated with using healthy individuals in a trial (which is not part of our discussion) but such subjects may represent a practical model in certain clinical pharmacology trials for the following reasons:

- *there is little variability* between individuals and this makes it possible to conduct conclusive trials with a limited number of subjects (statistical comparisons are all the more significant when differences between subjects are small);

- when administering a new agent to humans for the first time, there is *less risk* in healthy volunteers than in patients whose health is already compromised (provided that the trial is conducted in an institution where adequate facilities for intensive care are available).

Certainly, trials in healthy volunteers have little chance of providing information on *the therapeutic value* of a compound, but in many instances one cannot easily do without them, at least with respect to initial toxicity and pharmacokinetic studies in man.

The rules for selection of healthy volunteers in phase I trials are quite different, and consist of negative criteria:
- for example, exclusion of all patients with manifest disorders by using appropriate explorations,
- a subject should not have donated blood or recently participated in another trial (for reasons of safety).

2. SELECTING HOMOGENEOUS GROUPS

Patients selected for a trial will differ but they must be comparable on at least two counts: an approximately similar prognosis of spontaneous evolution of the disease during the trial, and an expected similar response to the treatments compared.

Indeed, a trial involving groups that are heterogeneous with regard to prognosis and treatment response might result in misleading conclusions:

• *the allocation of patients to several groups* (one per treatment) carries a high risk of non-comparability;

• *the variability of "responses"* to treatments would be increased, making statistical comparison less sensitive;

• *the conclusions of the trial* would not be sufficiently explicit for lack of precise definition of the type of patients to whom the results could be generalized;

• *an ambiguous definition* of the type of patient to be studied might lead to dissimilar patient recruitment and non-reproducible results.

Figure 1

Quantitative variable: if patients are selected on the basis of a value lying beyond an arbitrary limit, the distribution of values among the patients will be highly asymmetrical. Furthermore, there is a strong likelihood of observing "a regression towards the mean" on subsequent measurements in the same patients.

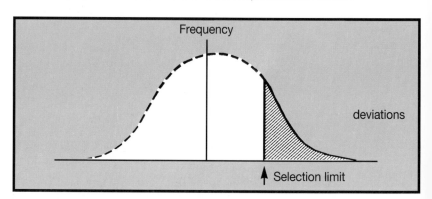

For these reasons, we must define with precision the following:

• *the operational definition* considered in the above paragragh: not only must the disorder be delimited with precision, but there is also the need for a certain degree of "narrowness". This often requires setting numerical limits for laboratory tests and describing how the tests are done and how the results are read.

If patients are selected on the basis of a quantitative variable (e.g. blood pressure, or blood sugar), and if the therapeutic result is evaluated by another measurement of the same variable, the phenomenon of "regression towards the true mean" must be considered.

Some subjects, for whom the mean value for a selection criterion lies below a given limit, are selected on the basis of the labile nature of this value (error by excess); similarly, other subjects, whose mean value lies above this limit, may be excluded definitively (selection error by default). Later these patient measurements return towards higher values, but they are no longer taken into account in the calculations for the sample recruited. This artifact explains the tendency of mean values "to return to normal" in successive measurements.

This difficulty arising from subjects who return spontaneously to a normal value before entering a trial may be avoided by successive measurements during a "run-in" period (10). However, it must be realized that the greater the number of measurements, the smaller the chance of retaining a patient who occasionally crosses the line separating normal and abnormal values. It has been suggested (4) that hypertensive patients might be tested on more than one occasion before entering the study using somewhat broader limits than the aim of the trial would imply (broadening the selection windows).

In general, comparisons are made more sensitive by including only subjects for whom successive measurements are *stable*. This can be achieved, for example, by defining the maximum tolerable deviation between two or more pretreatment measurements.

• *Concomitant disorders*: those disorders which may influence either the course of the disease under study, the evaluation criteria for the results, or the metabolic fate of the compounds being compared, must be excluded. It is for this reason, for example, that subjects with renal failure are often ineligible for a trial.

• *The physiological or demographic characteristics* of the patients may also influence the results of a trial and must be given due consideration. Some of the factors that may be important are age, gender, height, and weight (especially if fixed dosage is used), pregnancy, occupation, reliability in keeping appointments (it is generally specified that the trial will exclude patients who present a risk of being lost to follow-up, for example those whose occupation entails frequent travel or changing their address), and previous compliance with treatments.

It must be noted that the lack of homogeneity in characteristics that influence neither the course of the illness nor the treatment, as a rule, is unimportant... unless, of course, it is noticed later that such factors did exert a subtle influence that was not initially recognized!

3. SELECTING "REPRESENTATIVE" GROUPS

As we saw in the preceding chapter, true representativeness can only be obtained in a random sample. This is then a utopia-like goal in the context of clinical trials (3).

Selection of patients does not, therefore, result in true sampling since it necessarily entails a number of important non-random factors: choice the physician by the patient, acceptance of treatment and participation the trial, exclusion of certain patient categories (age, concomita disorders, etc.) Such factors strongly alter representativeness and v result in the groups having a different composition than that of tl "population".

One must reason by analogy and generalize results to subjects wi similar characteristics to those in the trial and treated under comparat conditions.

To obtain a reasonable generalization (phase 3), the recruitment mu then cover a *fairly broad spectrum* of the disease condition under stu (12, 17) and of the demographic categories of the population. particular, under-representation of women subjects in trials has oft been pointed out (6). If there is reason to believe that ethnic differenc may play a part, they must be taken into account in the program development (13, 15, 18). It is recommended to keep a screening lo book (4) in which all patients with the disorder under study, but exclud from the trial for whatever reason, will be recorded together with tl reason for their exclusion.

The requirements of homogeneity and representativeness a contradictory: the more "homogeneous" the group, the le "representative" it will be and a reasonable compromise is not alwa easy to find.

4. ASSURING REALISTIC RECRUITMENT

Experience has shown that before a trial, recruitment is *regular overestimated* (7). The illness, thought to be common, sudden "disappears" as soon as one starts looking for it and then seems reappear when the trial is over.

This phenomenon is often referred to as "Lasagna's law" and there are number of particularly demonstrative examples (1, 2, 5).

It can be explained by the necessarily rigorous criteria for eligibil related to the disease and by the elimination of many potenti participants who meet the entry criteria but who are ineligible based (exclusion criteria. Moreover, the enthusiasm of the investigators genera tends to decline and recruitment gradually diminishes if the trial extended for any length of time (11). Then too, drift away from stri selection towards broader recruitment during the trial is a comm temptation. This protocol violation changes the meaning of the tr results, to a greater or lesser extent.

Pilot studies are partly justified because they may help to evalua recruitment problems.

In some countries, it is possible to use techniques similar to marketir methods (newspaper advertisements, posters, radio announcements.. They are applicable only if regulations of the country so authorizes (1, 1

5. OBSERVING ETHICAL PRINCIPLES

Whenever the trial in itself or one of the compounds under study presents an unacceptable risk for the patient, he should be excluded from the trial. Of course, such risks must be weighed against those of the treatment that the patient would be receiving were he not a subject in the trial. This is the reason why, for example, a trial protocol will often exclude women who may be in the first trimester of pregnancy (owing to the unknown teratogenic potential of a new drug), or patients suffering from a chronic condition, that is well-controlled and in whom it would be necessary to interrupt effective treatment.

Except for the fairly uncommon situation in which slightly lesser efficacy of a treatment is temporarily acceptable (hypnotic drugs for example), one systematic criterion of eligibility might be "subjects for whom all the various treatments proposed for study are indicated".

6. DEFINING THE SELECTION CRITERIA

The trial protocol must include a precise and unambiguous definition of all the *eligibility criteria* as well as all *the exclusion criteria*.

6.1. Eligibility criteria

• The disorder to be studied must be precisely defined (and not simply named) and its nosologic limits specified (what will be done with "marginal" or "borderline" cases?). If several systems for classification of disease entities exist (in psychiatry for example), selection of one or the other can account for differences in results (7);

• The forms of the illness which are acceptable should be described (symptoms, etiology, course, including stage of the disease, complications, duration, factors liable to modify the course either favorably or unfavorably);

• The patient's characteristics must be clearly stated:
- age limits,
- sex,
- occupation and extra-curricular activities, psychological and linguistic factors, if relevant (if questioning the patient is important for evaluating the results);

• Consenting subjects.

6.2. Exclusion criteria

These include characteristics liable to jeopardize the evaluation of the results, or the safety of the treatments compared or the "faithfulness" of patients anticipated in complying with the protocol:

• unevaluable cases:
This category includes all subjects in whom it is anticipated that it will be difficult to obtain a correct evaluation, for example:

- subjects with linguistic difficulties in the case of self-rating or a questionnaire;
- a treadmill test for a subject with osteoarthritis of the hip ...;

• exclusions for safety reasons:
- contraindications to *one* of the treatments compared (list and define them);
- concomitant disorders (for example, renal failure which must be defined by precise criteria);
- concomitant medications that are not compatible with the drugs compared;
- pregnancy or possible pregnancy (no effective contraception) or even "women of child-bearing potential";

• exclusion of subjects expected to be "non compliant" to the protocol:
- subjects who have little chance of returning to see the physician on the required dates or unlikely to take the treatment as prescribed (no permanent address, unmotivated subjects).

7. POOR SELECTION CRITERIA

Relatively often, the results of a trial cannot be used because of recruitment criteria:
- too broad or too narrow selection,
- patients too sick or not sick enough,
- populations that are too particular,
- definition too vague or not reproducible.

References

1 Calimlim J, Wardell WM, Lasagna L. Selection, attrition and consent in the recruitment of patients for a clinical trial. Clin Pharmacol Ther 1977; *21*: 100.

2 Collins JF, Bingham SF, Weiss DG, Williford WO, Kuhn RM. Some adaptive strategies for inadequate sample acquisition in Veterans Administration cooperative trials. Controlled Clinical Trials 1980; *1*: 227-48.

3 Feinstein AR. Clinical Biostatistics. VII. The rancid sample, the tilted target, and the medical poll-bearer. Clin Pharmacol Ther 1971; *12*: 134-50.

4 Goldman A. Design of blood pressure screening for clinical trials of hypertension. J Chron Dis 1976; *29*: 613-24.

5 Hassar M, Weintraub M. "Uninformed" consent and the healthy volunteer: an analysis of patient volunteers in a clinical trial of a new anti-inflammatory drug. Clin Pharmacol Ther 1976; *20*: 379-86.

6 Kinney EL, Trautmann J, Gold JA, Vessel ES, Zelis R. Under-representation of women in new drug trials. Annals of Internal Medicine 1981; *95*: 495-9.

7 Leff JP. Influence of selection of patients on results of clinical trials. Br Med J 1973; *4*: 156-8.

8 Montgomery SA. Common errors in clinical trials. In: Diagnosis and treatment of depression. Paris: Medsi/McGraw Hill, 1987: 410.

9 Overall JE, Goldstein BJ, Brauzer S. Symptomatic volunteers in psychiatric research. J Psychiat Res 1971; *9*: 31-43.

10 Rosner B. Screening for hypertension - some statistical observations. J Chron Dis 1977; *30*: 7-18.

11 Sherry S. Clinical trials with antithrombotic and thrombolytic agents. Principles and pitfalls. Thrombos, Diathes Haemorrh. (Stutt.) 1973; *29*: 3-10.

12 Simon P. Patient heterogeneity in clinical trials. Cancer Treat Resp 1980; *64*: 405-10.

13 Svenson CK. Representation of American Blacks in clinical trials of new drugs. JAMA 1989; *261*: 263-5.

14 Swinehart JM. Patient recruitment and enrollment into clinical trials - A discussion of specific methods and disease states. J Clin Res Pharmacoepidemiology 1991; *5*: 35-47.

15 Venter CP, Joubert PH. Ethnic differences in responses to B1-adrenoreceptor blockade by propanolol. J Cardiovasc Pharmacol 1984; *6*: 361-4.

16 Wittenborn JR. Guidelines for clinical trials of psychotropic drugs. Pharmakopsychiatrie. Neuro-psychopharmakologie 1977; *10*: 205-31.

17 Yusuf S, Held P, Teu KK, Toretsky ER. Selection of patients for randomized controlled trials: implications of wide or narrow eligibility criteria. Statistics in Medicine 1990; *9*: 73-86.

18 Zhou HH, Koshakji RP, Silberstein DJ, Wilkinson GR, Wood AJJ. Racial differences in drug response. New England J Med 1989; *320*: 565-70.

4 - Efficacy assessment

SUMMARY

The efficacy of treatments compared in a clinical trial should be evaluated on the basis of the aim of the trial. Their main qualities are as follows:
- sensitivity (detection of small variations),
- specificity (no false positives),
- reproducibility of measurements (made by the same observer) and agreement of measurements (made by different observers).

Repeated measurements provide greater assurance of the stability and also permit monitoring of a symptom over a given period of time. Finally, certain specific difficulties encountered in special cases should be given due attention: overall patient preference, ranking techniques, self-rating and observer rating scales, therapeutic supplements, and composite indices.

The conclusions derived from a clinical trial will depend, among other factors, on the criteria used to assess the efficacy of the treatments compared. If multiple criteria are used, it should be decided in advance which one will be used as the basis for confirmatory analysis of the results.

1. CHOICE OF CRITERIA AS A FUNCTION OF THE OBJECTIVE

A distinction must be made between preventive, curative, symptomatic or palliative treatments.

1.1. Preventive treatment

The criterion of response for preventive treatment combines the incidence and the time of onset of the disease event for which prevention is expected. Prevention is termed *primary* if the patient has not previously been affected, as in the case of vaccination trials, and *secondary* if the aim is to prevent a relapse, as in recurrent myocardial infarction studies. The method used, analysis of survival rates is described in chapter 15.

The application of the criterion of disease incidence requires accurate definition of the disease entity and strict, albeit arbitrary, limits must be set for borderline cases when relevant.

It is also necessary to accurately describe the methods of assessment used so that the chances of detection are the same from one patient to another and from one group to another (operational definitions).

Finally, a *follow-up period* must be set during which all patients in the trial will be monitored for signs of the disease under consideration. The length of the follow-up period depends on the rate of appearance of the disease entity: extended period of observation, limited only by material constraints of the trial investigators.

1.2. Curative treatment

Generally, the aim of curative treatment is to shorten the course of an acute disorder or to prevent an unfavorable outcome. The criterion of response is therefore either:

- the duration of the disease, which sometimes requires definition of the limit between the "ill" state and the state of "recovery";

- or the incidence of complications or fatal outcome.

1.3. Symptomatic treatment

Generally, symptomatic treatment aims to alleviate a symptom without claiming to influence the course of the underlying disease. The criteria of response assess either the *severity* of the symptom by using a quantitative scale of clinical manifestations to define the extent of improvement, or the *duration* of the effect obtained, or the *incidence* of episodes during a defined time period.

1.4. Palliative treatment

The purpose of palliative treatment is to delay an inescapable outcome (generally death). As with preventive treatment, the criterion of response is the *time that elapses* before the endpoint under study is reached. The duration of follow-up from the start of treatment is not necessarily the same for all patients. It is taken into account by using what is called the "life-table method" which is discussed in another chapter. This method is preferable to individual estimates such as the rate of onset of the endpoint after a given time period (e.g. 5-year survival) and the mean time or median time which elapses between the start of treatment and the occurrence of the event (e.g. median duration of survival).

1.5. Other criteria

Finally, the main criterion for comparing treatments is not always therapeutic efficacy. In some cases the criterion may be tolerability, patient acceptability or the incidence of withdrawals (during prolonged treatments).

2. THE CONCEPT OF "MEASUREMENT"

Measuring a variable means comparing it to a known standard defined as a "unit" and then determining how many such units it contains. A measurement is meaningful only within certain *limits of uncertainty* determined by the *accuracy* of the method used. Indeed, accidental errors in measurement may distort the result. The smaller the errors in measurement, the more sensitive the statistical comparisons.

Changing units simply comes down to either multiplying the result by a constant (e.g. transforming classical laboratory units into SI units) or doing it after addition or subtraction of a 2nd constant (e.g. conversion of Fahrenheit temperature to Celsius). The same transformation constants apply to the mean and to the standard deviation. Thus, altering units has *no bearing on the significance of statistical tests*.

The actual physical operation of measurement (e.g. reading a value from a dial) is often associated with a "digit preference" error that subconsciously tends to give preference to "round" numbers (ending in 0 or 5) or "even" numbers.This tendency can be corrected when the operator is aware of it and thus improve the precision of the measurement.

Conversely, some types of apparatus may express the result using a number of digits that is meaningless given the overall degree of accuracy of the measurement. The results are then usually *"rounded off"* by eliminating the excess digits. It is, however, necessary to maintain enough digits to express deviation from the mean by at least two digits. Even imprecise measurements should not be merged into broader classes since the resultant *loss of information* is prejudicial to the sensitivity of the statistical comparison (even if it simplifies the calculations).

3. VALUES OR INADEQUACIES OF ASSESSMENT CRITERIA

3.1. "Objective" or "subjective" criteria

The appealing distinction between objective and subjective criteria is usually not as clear-cut as may be imagined. Admittedly, symptoms such as pain or anxiety do not lend themselves to "physical" measurement, while at the other end of the scale an automated laboratory test appears to eliminate the problem of subjective interpretation. There is, nevertheless, virtually always a subjective component in all "objective" measurements and we must thus recognize that errors in measurement are more often made unconsciously to suit the investigator's preferences rather than in any other direction (13). Moreover, some tests may appear to be "objective" because they are derived through technical means (X-ray or electrocardiogram) but they require interpretation which involves a subjective element, as shown by the differences in interpretation when the results of apparently objective tests are read by several different persons (8, 30).

Rechecking measurements that produce questionable (i.e. aberrant) results also introduces an arbitrary component into the most "objective" measurement since this means having a different attitude towards *expected results*, which are not verified, and *unexpected results* which are. A precise limit between the two is generally not defined beforehand. This approach often leads to eliminating "errors" which deviate markedly from the mean and not those which come close to it.

Finally, objectivity is *wrongly* considered to be an advantage when an attempt is made to achieve it by substituting an indirect criterion for assessing a highly subjective one with which it is weakly correlated. For example, an electrodermal test in anxious subjects does not provide much information on what sensation they really feel.

3.2. Direct or indirect criteria - validation

Generally, the aim of a treatment is not to improve some laboratory test result in patients. Erythrocyte sedimentation rate, which is only weakly linked to *clinical* improvement in rheumatoid arthritis, can hardly be chosen as the major criterion for testing an anti-inflammatory agent.

The only reason for reducing blood pressure in hypertensive patients is that we know that this reduces mortality and morbidity. In the treatment of hypertension, the direct criterion is the incidence of complications. Measurement of blood pressure is therefore an indirect criterion in this case.

If the indirect criterion has been proved to be strongly linked to the direct criterion, the former can be used as a surrogate endpoint (23).

Moreover, when a *new test* is used to assess the severity of a disease entity, the problem of its validation must be established *before* it can be used in a clinical trial. To do this, it must be shown that its results are "strongly correlated" with those of the old method.

3.3. Errors in measurement, metrological properties

For a given assessment criterion, it is useful to identify all causes of error by classifying them into four categories: those which are due:
- to the instrument (questionnaire or apparatus): they may be prevented by standardization,
- to the method of use of the instrument: they may be prevented by providing a detailed method of operation (specific operating procedure),
- to the rater: these can be limited by training sessions,
- to the patient: these can be prevented by not including subjects who are difficult to evaluate.

There are two types of differences between the results of measurements and actual values:

- systematic errors by constant or progressive over- or underestimations,
- random, unforeseeable errors, around true values which increase the variance of results.

These two types of errors condition the properties of measurements.

3.3.1. Sensitivity

An assessment criterion is sensitive if it can detect minor improvements or deteriorations in a condition.

A sensitivity criterion is often a quantitative one and this sometimes means mistakenly choosing a *measurable but indirect criterion that will show up small variations*. The result is a *risk of compromising validity for the sake of sensitivity.*

It is also important that the sensitivity of a new criterion be established before a negative result based on that criterion can be accepted. The fact that no difference was shown between the treatments compared may be related to the inability of the measurement to demonstrate a real difference if one exists.

3.3.2. Repeatability

This is the consistency of results obtained by the same observer operating under the same conditions in a short time span.

3.3.3. Reproducibility

This is the consistency of results obtained by different observers at different times. Agreement of two observers measuring the same criterion is called "concordance".

It is preferable that measurements always be made by the *same observer*, who should be *trained* in observing and in minimizing his own observer error. In addition, observer error can sometimes be reduced by having two or more observers make the measurements.

3.3.4. Specificity

By *specificity* is meant that a criterion is not influenced by variables other than those which one seeks to measure. Specificity is often contradicting with sensitivity since as the latter increases, smaller and smaller differences show up, but the risk of detecting known or unsuspected artifacts also increases.

3.4. Stability

A measurable criterion is said to be *stable* if it does not fluctuate "too widely" from one recording to another in the same individual. Otherwise it is said to be *labile*.

Stability can be improved by standardizing measurement techniques and the conditions that may affect them, such as the time of day, environmental, temperature and physiological circumstances...

For overly labile variables, a relatively "stable" reading can be obtained by taking the mean of several measurements performed during the same examination. For example, it is recommended that blood pressure recordings be repeated two or three times after completely deflating the cuff between each recording.

In some chronic conditions it may be relevant to take account of *seasonal variations* in evaluating treatment outcome. Examples include angina pectoris, intermittent claudication, rheumatic disorders and depressive illness. This can be achieved in several ways:

- by restricting patient recruitment to a single season or even, if possible by recruiting all the patients at the same time and following them up synchronously;

- by balancing the treatment groups on the basis of seasonal recruitment;

- by recording the dates of entry of all patients so as to at least permit verification of group comparability after the end of the study.

4. REPEATED MEASUREMENTS AND THEIR CHRONOLOGY

4.1. Measurement before and after treatment (13, 15)

When the criterion of response is the variation in a measurement or in the severity of a symptom, it should be evaluated before and after treatment and the effect analyzed:

• either the *absolute difference*, which places equal importance on a given change, regardless of initial values;

• or the relative difference or *percent change* which places greater importance on a given change if the initial score is low;

• or on the basis of the value after treatment *adjusted* for "equal pretreatment values" (for example, analysis of covariance or analysis stratified by initial scores).

These modalities will be dealt with in the chapter on analysis of results. Interpreting results is sometimes difficult or even impossible if the mean pretreatment values differ substantially between the groups compared. Figure 1 shows three examples.

It is not always possible to "compensate" adequately for pretreatment differences, particularly if the differences subsequently observed between the groups are only "marginally significant".

4.2. Repeated measurements before treatment

Repeat measurements during a more or less prolonged pretreatment period provide a more accurate reflection of the baseline status if the criterion of response is a labile one. Common examples include measurement of blood pressure and rating scales in psychiatry.

Figure 1
"Before" and "after"
measurements. Interpretation
of three difficult cases.

The initial difference probably
contributes to the final
difference.

The pretreatment difference
may mask the difference in
efficacy.

This result cannot be
interpreted clearly and will
have only token value.

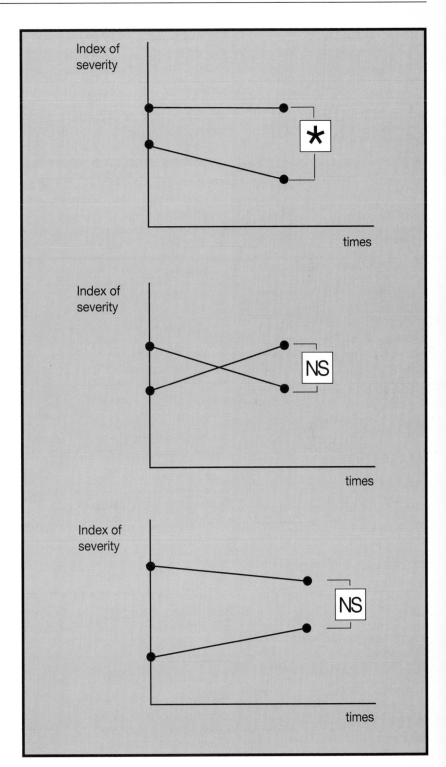

4.3. Repeated measurements during treatment

Repeating measurements during the treatment period allows evaluation of the change in the criterion under the effect of treatment. We then speak of the influence of the "time" factor and "time-treatment" interaction. In this case the analysis of the results must use a global method for "repeated measurements" and not separate repeated tests which raise the possibility of finding a significant result by chance alone. In practice, if there is no time-treatment interaction, then the curves representing the effect of each treatment will be parallel. In other cases, the treatments differ in the rapidity or duration of effect.

Figure 2 shows a few examples of time-effect curves, with or without time-treatment interaction, and figure 3 illustrates some schematic cases of time-treatment interactions. It can be noted on some of these curves how erroneous or incomplete the conclusions of a trial can be if the observation period is too short or if there are no intermediate values correctly recorded.

A crucial problem is the choice of timing for measurements which should take account of the kinetics of the treatment effect, nycthemeral variations in the variable measured, and the practical feasibility.

It is important to point out, moreover, that when the number of patients is small, *fluctuations with time* may be substantial and may mask the general pattern of the time-effect relationship, or simulate peaks or intersections on the curves. Consequently, only a significant interaction allows to conclude that there is a *difference in the time-course*.

In some trials (single-dose antihypertensive drugs taken once daily), a major criterion is the residual effect before the next dose is taken (26).

It is also possible to simplify a succession of repeated measurements by reducing them to *the mean of the measurements* for each subject or to their sum provided that the same number of measurements were made for each subject. During clinical trials on analgesics (1, 4, 29), the sum of differences between initial pain score and later scores is often used.

5. SPECIAL CASES

5.1. Preference between two treatment periods

When two treatments are administered successively to the same patients, each patient may be asked which treatment he preferred and the number of preferences for each treatment can then be compared. The advantage of this approach is that it gives an overall view, taking into account both efficacy and tolerability, with the relative importance that each patient implicitly and subconsciously attributes to each of these factors. It may be ambiguous, however, and should not be used if a short-term benefit perceived by the patient (or a pleasant or euphoric effect), masks a harmful long-term effect or a disadvantage of which only the investigator is aware.

Figure 2

Schematic representation of the
effects of treatment, time and
the time x treatment interaction
(parallel group design)
S = index of severity
T = effect of treatment
t = effect of time
t x T = time x treatment
interaction

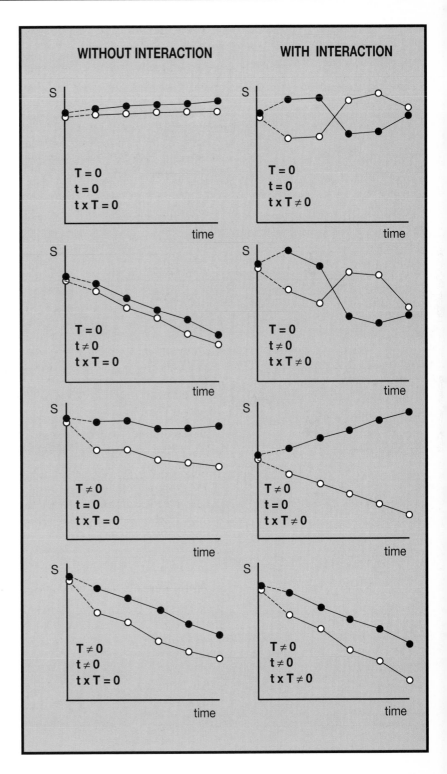

45

Figure 3
Examples of interpretation of time-treatment interaction.

Top to bottom: difference in
- rapidity of effect,
- duration of effect,
- rapidity and duration,
- curves which intersect indicate that one treatment is more effective early (O) and the other more effective later (●)

S = index of severity

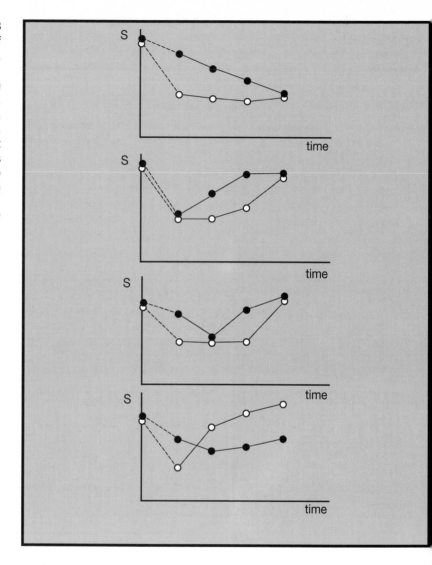

For this reason, it is wiser to consider both the "patient's preference" and the "physician's preference", the latter often being based on very different criteria which should be clearly defined, if possible.

Furthermore, the statistical methods used to compare the number of preferences for each treatment generally disregard cases where the subject says he cannot decide (ties). This may be problematical if the number of "no opinions" is substantial or if patients are "forced" into expressing a preference that may have no real clinical significance.

5.2. Ranking subjects

If a non-quantitative but comparable permanently recorded criterion can be obtained from all patients, they can be classified *a posteriori* in order of severity for the same criterion before and after treatment. The respective rank of each patient who received the drugs tested can then be compared.

This procedure has been advocated (12) to classify handwriting samples from patients with Parkinson's disease ranked in order of the degree of alteration.

5.3. Self-rating scales

Some symptoms, essentially those that are subjective (pain, fatigue), can be assessed only by the patient himself. Several techniques can be used to refine the patients' answers:

• A visual analogue scale, consisting of a horizontal or vertical line, generally 10 cm long, each end of which represents an extreme state for the criterion under consideration, defined by appropriate opposing words or phrases (figure 4). The patient is asked to situate his status somewhere between these two extremes. It is preferable not to mark intermediate reference points on such a scale as this clearly influences the patients' responses which tend to lose their uniform distribution and cluster around the reference points (17). It is generally not advisable to allow patients to see their preceding score at the time of a subsequent rating.

Some patients give aberrant answers and it may be useful to exclude them during a pre-test period (20).

Figure 4
Visual analogue scales

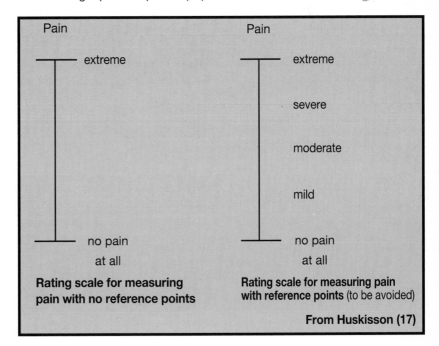

• A choice of adverbs: a questionnaire with several possible ready-made answers can be put to the patient who is asked to choose only one. In practice, this generally comes down to choosing among a list of adverbs qualifying frequency ("often", "rarely"...) or severity ("moderately", "markedly"...).

In this case, the adverbs used should have been tested from a psychological standpoint for their order, for example in a prior sample of volunteers (if possible fairly similar to the trial participants from the ethnic, linguistic and sociocultural standpoints) (2, 5).

Selecting the most appropriate number of choices is important since too few choices will not permit a sufficiently fine classification and too many will introduce overly subtle distinctions that may confuse the subject.

• Finally, self-rating scales may be *absolute* (i.e. the patient is asked to record the severity of a symptom) or *relative* (i.e. degree of improvement or worsening).

The latter is more sensitive since it eliminates the effect of the variability of the initial status (16). However, unlike "absolute" rating, "relative" rating *cannot be repeated*, since it is difficult for the patient to distinguish the degree of improvement in comparison to baseline or in comparison to the last rating made.

Finally, self-rating necessarily implies three conditions: comprehension of the instructions by the patient, cooperation of the patient and careful checking of the answers by the clinician.

5.4. "Symptomatic" or "Supplementary" treatments

Symptomatic treatments are additional to long-term treatment and on which it is desired to assess their effects: e.g. Nitroglycerin consumption in patients with angina pectoris, analgesics in those with rheumatic disease. This procedure has the advantage of not depriving the patient of a treatment that may alleviate his or her symptoms without hindering the assessment of the long-term treatment. Its major drawback is the variability in the motivation of patients taking the symptomatic treatment: habit, prevention, or for variable degrees of pain or discomfort.

Moreover, it is conceivable that a long-term treatment that has no effect per se may potentiate the therapeutic efficacy of the symptomatic treatment, thus reducing its consumption by two different mechanisms. Clinical interpretation can be difficult in these trials if one group has both lower consumption together with lower efficacy.

5.5. Composite indices (6, 7)

Some diseases present multiple symptoms and one may not wish to select a single one of these as the only criterion of response but rather consider several symptoms simultaneously to permit overall assessment of the efficacy of a treatment. This may be done by adding the scores of severity for each individual symptom, with the option of attributing different weights to each symptom. Arbitrary weights can be replaced by weights extracted from the statistical technique known as a principal components analysis (21). It must be kept in mind however, that these "factors" are obtained from the maximum variance criterion which is a statistical criterion and has no greater *clinical* validity than arbitrarily chosen weights.

The most common example is that of indices used to evaluate the inflammatory syndrome in rheumatic diseases (6, 19, 24). Composite indices have been accused of being arbitrary, of having obscure clinical significance or of not being validated for the underlying inflammatory or other process. Nonetheless, they have proved their empirical value for evaluating the efficacy of treatments in these patients.

In any case, composite indices can only be used if the decision to do so is made *before* commencing the trial, otherwise one can readily conceive of using all sorts of indices, *a posteriori*, more or less validated and of only retaining the "most favorable" one.

5.6. Rating scales comprising multiple items (11, 13, 14)

Rating scales are used to standardize the evaluation of a syndrome expressed more or less directly by clinical manifestations or items. The severity of each item is rated using a self-rating questionnaire or by ratings made by an experienced and qualified rater.

The design and use of rating scales raise specific problems that cannot be dealt with in detail in this book (25).

Scales are used primarily in psychiatry studies (scales for depression, anxiety, etc) but questionnaires for evaluating sleep (16, 22, 25), appetite (9) and other symptoms have also been used. When several possible scales are available for studying a particular syndrome, the choice should be made after consulting the literature and specialized books (3, 10, 28) for the following points:

- the mode of use: standardization of a classical history, self-rating questionnaires filled out by the patient (easy-to-use but preclude interpretation on the basis of information provided by an observer, also not applicable to severely ill patients or those with linguistic problems), or recording of the patient's behavior, by a member of the nursing staff for example;

- the exact significance of the items and the definition of the grades (often multiple choice questions relating to the frequency or severity of a symptom). It must also be ensured that none of the items is absurd or irrelevant to the population and the context studied;

- the method for calculating the overall score (simple sum of individual scores, weighted sum or partial score derived from a group of items) and the values generally obtained in healthy and sick subjects. The "additive" hypothesis (postulating that equal global scores obtained by adding-up different item scores are equivalent) is a useful but rough simplification of reality.

- the validity: proportionality between the score and the severity of the symptom assessed in some other way and the aptitude to differentiate the treatments compared in the trial;

- the training that may be necessary to obtain reliable scores. One must be aware of systematic *tendencies* to attribute scores that are either too high or too low (extreme tendencies) or too "average" (central effect) or to attribute similar scores to adjacent items (halo effect).

It is recommended that a scale should not be modified unless its validity has been verified again and not to use a new scale in a trial unless its results are checked against a classical scale.

5.7 Regularity of the effect

In some situations, the aim of the study may be to demonstrate a difference in the consistency of effect between two treatments rather than a difference in the mean effect.

This implies designing a trial in which the effect in each patient comes as close as possible to the mean effect (particularly by dosage adjustment) and then comparing the *variances* of the treatment effects.

This procedure may be of use when the reproducibility of effects is an advantage, particularly if the bioavailability of the treatments compared is different (improved bioavailability resulting in less variable effects) (18) or for comparing sustained-release preparations of the same drug where greater regularity of the sustained-effect is considered as an advantage.

In other circumstances, a greater variance with one of the treatments might be due to the existence of a subgroup of "non-responders" which it will be useful to describe later.

References

1   Calimlim JF, Wardell WM, Lasagna L, Gillies AJ, Davis HT. Effect of naloxone on the analgesic activity of methadone in 1: 10 oral combination. Time and cost of flirting with the null hypothesis in tests of equivalence. Clin Pharmacol Ther 1974; *15*: 556-664.

2   Cliff N. Adverbs as multipliers. Psychol Rev 1959; *66*: 27-44.

3   Collegium Internationale Psychiatrie Scalarum. Internationale Skalen für Psychiatrie. Frankfurt: Hoechst AG, 1977.

4   Cooper SA, Beaver WT. A model to evaluate mild analgesics in oral surgery outpatients. Clin Pharmacol Ther 1976; *20*: 214-50.

5   Delay J, Pichot P, Perse J. Note sur la sélection d'adverbes d'intensité et de fréquence dans la construction d'épreuves psychométriques. Rev Psychol Appl 1964; *14*: 169-78.

6   Eberl R. Summation devices are useful. In: Paulus HE, Erlich GE, Lindenlaub E, eds. Controversies in the clinical evaluation of analgesic-anti-inflammatory-anti-rheumatic drugs. Stuttgart: Schattauer Verlag, 1980.

7   Feinstein AR. Clinical biostatistics, IX. How do we measure "safety and efficacy"? Clin Pharmacol Ther 1971; *1*: 544-58.

8   Feinstein AR, Kramer MS. Clinical biostatistics, LIII. The architecture of the observer/method variability and other types of process research. Clin Pharmacol Ther 1980; *28*: 551-63.

9   Gagnon MA, Tetreault L. Pharmacologie humaine des anorexigènes. Validité d'un questionnaire sur l'appétit. Union Médicale du Canada 1975; *104*: 922-9.

10 Guy W. ECDEU. Assessment manual for psycho-pharmacology. Rockville: NIMH, 1976.

11 Guyatt GH. Measuring quality of life: a review of means of measurement in clinical trials of medicines. Pharmaceut Med 1987; *2*: 49-60.

12 Hamilton M. Measurement in medicine. Lancet 1958; *i*: 982-97.

13 Hamilton M. Lectures on the methodology of clinical research. Edinburgh: Churchill Livingstone 1974; 126.

14 Hamilton M. Measurement in psychiatry. In: Van Praag HM, ed. Handbook of biological psychiatry. New York: Marcel Dekker, 1979.

15 Hill GB. The statistical analysis of clinical trials. Br J Anaesth 1967; *39*: 294-314.

16 Hindmarch I. A 1-4 Benzodiazepine, Temazepam (K 3917), its effects on some psychological parameters of sleep behaviour. Arzneim Forsch 1975; *25*: 1836-39.

17 Huskisson EC. Measurement of pain. Lancet 1974; *2*: 1127-31.

18 Imbs JL, Schmidt M, Spriet A, Schwartz J. Variance as a tool in clinical pharmacology: an example with two loop diuretics. Europ J Clin Pharmacol 1982; *22*: 222-5.

19 Lansbury J. Methods for evaluating rheumatoid arthritis. In: Arthritis and allied conditions. Hollander JL, McCarthy DJ, eds. 6th ed. Lea and Febiger 1972: 250-73.

20 Lewis RV, Jackson PR, Ramsay LE. Visual analogue scales for side-effects of beta-adrenoreceptor blocking drugs: reproducibility of scoring. Pharmaceut Med 1987; *1*: 273-8.

21 McGuire RJ, Wright V. Statistical approach to a trial of Indomethacin. Ann Rheum Dis 1971; *30*: 574-80.

22 Parrott AC, Hindmarch I. Factor analysis of a sleep evaluation questionnaire. Psychol Med 1978; *8*: 325-9.

23 Prentice RL. Surrogate endpoints in clinical trials: definition and operational criteria. Statistics in Medicine 1989; *8*: 331-40.

24 Ritchie DM, Boyle JA, McInnes JM et al. Clinical studies with an articular index for the assessment of joint tenderness in patients with rheumatoid arthritis. Quar J Med 1968; *37*: 393-406.

25 Spriet A, Fermanian J. Les échelles d'évaluation en psychopharmacologie. L'Encéphale 1978; *4*: 119-29.

26 Stewart WH, Hafner KB. Statistical analysis of trough/peak ratios. Drug Information Journal 1991; *25*: 405-9.

27 Sundaresan PR, Wardell WM, Weintraub M, Lasagna L. Methodology for demonstrating sustained efficacy of hypnotics: a comparative study of triazolam and flurazepam. Clin Pharmacol Ther 1979; *25*: 391-8.

28 Van Riezen H, Segal M. Comparative evaluation of rating scales for clinical psychopharmacology. Amsterdam: Elsevier, 1988.

29 Weintraub M, Jacox RF, Angevine CD, Atwater EC. Piroxicam (CP 1617) in rheumatoid arthritis: a controlled clinical trial with novel assessment techniques. J Rheumatol 1977; *4*: 393-404

30 Yerushalmy J, Harkness JT, Cope JH, Kennedy BR. The role of dual reading in mass radiography. Amer Rev Tuberculosis 1950; *61*: 443-64.

5 - Randomization

SUMMARY

Assignment of patients to treatment groups by randomization is the only way to insure that the assigned treatment cannot be predicted at the time of patient selection, that the treatment is independent of the patient's characteristics and that uncontrolled variability factors are distributed at random between the groups. In practice, tables of random numbers are used (or better still tables of random permutations which periodically balance the number of patients in each group) or algorithms which simulate these random numbers in computer calculations.

Stratification enables separate randomization within subsets of patients with comparable prognosis. This procedure permits broader recruitment of patients but it is limited by the number of prognostic factors that can be used.

Finally, adaptive procedures for treatment assignment can be used either to balance the distribution of prognostic factors as the trial proceeds, or to assign a progressively increasing number of patients to the treatment which stands out as the most effective.

In a controlled trial, patients must be subdivided into as many groups as there are therapeutic regimens to be compared. Allocating subjects to groups is done by random allocation. This procedure is justified on theoretical and practical grounds and several methods are available.

1. RANDOM ASSIGNMENT

1.1. Justification

True random assignment is the only procedure that assures the unpredictability and independence of patient assignment to treatment groups, and consistency with the laws of probability upon which statistical tests are based.

1.1.1. Unpredictability

The unpredictable nature of randomization (10) means that it is impossible to know which treatment any given patient will receive. Thus, one is certain not to orient decisions on patients eligibility according to the treatments that they are going to receive.

No other treatment assignment technique (e.g. alternative allocation, odd and even days, birth date, first letter of the patient's name, etc.) has the same advantage of avoiding treatment assignment predictability (1,18)

1.1.2. Independence between treatment assignment and results

Randomization is the only procedure for which it can be stated with certainty that treatment is in no way related to the characteristics of the patient or the severity of the prognosis, and thus indirectly with the results of treatment. In other words, randomization avoids bias in assigning patients to treatment groups. The other conceivable procedures all suffer from a potential direct or indirect relationship (sometimes subtle) with chances of treatment success.

Obvious examples include:

• using patients who are ineligible for, or who refuse treatment A to form a group which receives treatment B;

• using non-concurrent series ("historical" controls or series drawn from "data banks") (3);

• comparing different treatments given by different investigators.

1.1.3. Consistency of randomization with probability theory

This very important reason is the least obvious justification for random assignment: all statistical tests postulate chance distribution of unpredictable variations (residual error) and of *uncontrolled* factors (it is impossible to control all the variables).

The only way to ensure that this distribution is really governed by chance alone is to use randomization. However, randomization does not eliminate the need for verifying *a posteriori* that the groups are comparable (30) within a "reasonable" number of comparisons on variables that are really liable to influence the results of the trial (19).

1.2. Randomization techniques

1.2.1. Simple techniques for random assignment

* The Japanese Standards Association (1-24 Akasanka 4, Minato-Ku, Tokyo 107 Japan) provides sets of three 20-sided, different color dice for this purpose.

Randomization may be performed by using a mechanical device such as a roulette wheel, dice*, "heads or tails" with a coin, or ballots drawn from a hat. It is less picturesque and more convenient to use tables of random numbers such as those of Fisher and Yates (15), which were originally drawn up using a random procedure. Furthemore, these tables have been tested to eliminate aberrant series (systematic progression, repetitive numbers, etc.) and to ensure that each figure appears the same number of times on the average.

An allocation rule is defined establishing a correspondance between each treatment and certain figures: for example, if we are comparing two treatments A and B it may be decided that:

0, 1, 2, 3 or 4 = treatment A
5, 6, 7, 8 or 9 = treatment B

If the series of numbers in the table begins by 279354008, this means that the first, fourth, sixth, seventh, and eight patients will receive treatment A and the second, third, fifth and ninth patients will receive treatment B.

If three treatments are being compared, it may be decided that:

1-2-3 = first treatment
4-5-6 = second treatment
7-8-9 = third treatment
(the zero is disregarded in this case)

When using tables of random numbers, figures must *always be read in the same direction*, say from left to right and from top to bottom. For successive trials, and even more so for the same trial, using the same part of the table several times over must be avoided.

In practice, computer-generated random numbers are useful for randomization of large groups of subjects, while making sure that the program does not always repeat the same series, either when starting up, or periodically (32).

1.2.2. Random permutations

Chance sometimes deals bad results:
- one treatment is assigned more often than another (producing unequal groups),
- or one treatment is given with greater frequency at the beginning of a trial and another with greater frequency at the end of the trial (this would result in time imbalance or chronological bias which is undesirable). To overcome this drawback, randomization may be performed in small batches or "blocks", each one comprising balanced number of each treatment.

To do this, a table of random permutations is used containing, in random order, all possible combinations (permutations) of a small series of figures.

With four figures, there are 1 x 2 x 3 x 4 = 24 possible combinations: 2314, 4312, 1423 … that are used with an allocation rule such as in the above.

In practice, the tables contain 6, 8, 10, 16 or 20 blocks of numbers. The same *predetermined direction* (for example always from top to bottom or left to right) must always be used.

Permutation series that are too short (2 or 4) and which enable prediction of treatment for at least the last patient if a partial code-break took place in a "non-blind" study must be avoided. Series which are too long risk producing unequal numbers of patients should recruitment stop in the middle of a series and must be avoided. Finally, permutation series of unequal length can be inserted to make the treatments more predictable.

1.2.3. Special cases

• If the subjects in a trial are to receive several treatments in a *different order* (within patient or crossover trial) the order in which they are administered must be determined randomly: AB or BA if the trial involves two treatments. Some experimental designs (latin square, incomplete block) require special randomization procedures which will be dealt with later.

• In some instances, there may be a need for unequal groups for the following reasons:

- a control group is compared with several treatments. To obtain optimal power for the statistical tests, the number of subjects is increased by a factor approximately equal to the square root of the number of treatments (9);

- in a placebo-controlled trial, the aim is to acquire more experience with the active drug. To obtain the same power as with equal numbers of subjects, the total number of cases must be increased in proportion to the imbalance desired. This increase is only 12.5% in the case of a 2 for 1 randomization.

• Zelen (36) has devised a procedure for comparing a proven treatment, assumed not to require patient consent, with a new treatment for which consent is deemed necessary. For the latter only, consent is requested and patients who refuse automatically receive the standard treatment *but remain in the "new treatment" group* for analysis of results. The justification for this approach lies in the fact that the comparison could be biased if the groups actually compared differed from those designated by the randomization procedure. However, if the number of refusals is substantial, the difference between treatment groups is diminished and the comparison will not be very sensitive.
Moreover, this procedure can only be applied to non-blind randomized trials. Finally, it does not solve the problem of consent from patients receiving the standard treatment but who, to fulfill the trial protocol requirements, must undergo more laboratory tests or procedures than dictated by standard care of their illness or who may complain that the new treatment was not proposed to them (22).

1.3. Timing of randomization

The randomization process should be prepared *in advance* and the predetermined list of treatment will serve to prepare the numbered drug containers (used *in order*) and the envelopes to be opened in case of an emergency.

When a new patient enters the study:

- if the trial is "blind", the patient should be given a number and his treatment assigned *at the last possible* moment when he has definitively been entered. (In this case, the envelopes are intended to be opened in case of an emergency).

- if the trial is not "blind", the envelope is opened *for assigning treatment*. There is a risk of bias if the envelopes are not numbered, if they are not used in the predetermined order or if any means whatever (transillumination) are used to guess what is inside or if an envelope is opened in advance. This has actually happened.

Remote allocation (telephone conversation, a voice frequency telephone connected to a computer information server...) after irreversible recording of the patient's identification makes it possible to overcome these drawbacks (5, 6, 24).

2. STRATIFICATION

If the groups formed by the randomization procedure were drawn from a *perfectly homogeneous "population"* (12), one could postulate that they were perfectly comparable, but this is rarely the case. Even after screening potential participants to ensure that they meet the selection criteria, we can still expect that the course of the disease will be more favorable in some patients for reasons independent of the treatment received, due to different "prognostic factors". Very "narrow" selection criteria may eliminate the influence of prognostic factors but it also considerably reduces recruitment and limits the generalizability of the results.

One can, of course, hope that chance alone will distribute prognostic factors evenly between randomly assigned groups and if this does not happen, any remaining disparities may simply *increase the variance* in the results and thus diminish the statistical sensitivity of the comparison without invalidating it.

Chance alone, however, may distribute prognostic factors unevenly (30) all the more so when the number of participants is small, thus introducing an important difference not due to treatments. When such a mishap occurs, separate analysis of comparable subgroups can still be performed retrospectively or adjusted to correct this discrepancy (2, 13).

But this "post-stratification" is somewhat arbitrary since the results observed may influence the way the groups are subdivided. Indirectly this comes down to formulating a hypothesis after examining the results and then testing the same results for statistical significance.

It is preferable to achieve balanced randomization *a priori* by randomizing within subgroups of patients who have comparable prognoses, also called *strata* (25). To describe this procedure, we shall successively consider the boundaries of strata, randomization of strata, the advantages and drawbacks of stratification.

2.1. Defining the boundaries of strata (2, 14)

The choice of strata may be based on a qualitative variable (e.g. sex) or a quantitative variable (e.g. blood pressure). In the latter case, the limit between two adjacent strata must be clearly defined:

e.g. diastolic blood pressure, measured under well-specified conditions:

- less than 100 mm Hg,
- greater than or equal to 100 and less than 110 mm Hg,
- etc.

The limits between strata should be chosen with the following points in mind:

• the subdivision should be based on variables that really have a bearing on the outcome of treatment. It is pointless to stratify for *a physiological* or sociodemographic *variable* (age, sex, intelligence, profession) if there is no reason to suspect that this variable might cause the treatment to have a different effect on the evaluation criterion chosen. The variables chosen therefore depend essentially on the disease entity under study and on what is known about its favorable or unfavorable prognostic factors (2);

• the strata must be mutually exclusive. There should be no ambiguity whatever as to which subgroup a given patient belongs, even if the limit between the two subgroups is arbitrary. If two subgroups overlap, a new stratum must be formed;

• two different strata must be *sufficiently discriminant*, that is they should correspond to assumedly different prognostic groups in which the results are expected to be different;

• each stratum must be homogeneous with regard to the efficacy of the treatments compared.

If the last two requirements are not adequately met, the limit between two adjacent strata may be changed for further trials by either combining two insufficiently discriminant strata, further subdivision of a heterogeneous stratum or rearrangement (displacing the limits separating adjacent strata).

• The limits between strata should be clearly defined so as to be reproducible in subsequent trials.

2.2. Multiple stratification (8, 14)

If several important prognostic factors have to be taken into account simultaneously, one of the following approaches may be used:

• stratification may be performed independently for each factor, but this quickly increases the number of subgroups (for example, stratification for two factors, say age and sex, produces 4 subgroups, but if stratification is performed for 4 factors, the number of subgroups rises to 16...);

• certain subgroups may be combined to form classes of comparable prognosis. Feinstein (14) for example considered blood pressure (3 subgroups) and serum cholesterol levels (3 subgroups) to form only 5 subgroups (classes A, B, C, D and E) instead of 9 theoretical subgroups using the following schema (figure 1):

Figure 1

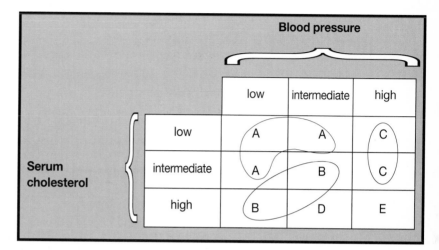

- strata may also be defined by several variables simultaneously, as in the classical definition of disease stages in cancer which includes local-regional extension, lymph node involvement and the presence or absence of distant metastases.

Composite indices defined by multiple variances to which different "weights" are assigned may also be used depending on their prognostic importance.

The choice of variables, weights and limits of strata must be justified by their relation with the course of the illness.

2.3. Randomization within strata

Within each stratum, patients should be allocated to treatment groups by randomization as described previously. As a rule, investigators rarely know in advance how many patients will be included in each stratum. Since randomization has to be prepared in advance, a surplus of patients should be anticipated to allow for the case where the recruitment in any given stratum exceeds expectations.

2.4. Advantages of stratification

The advantages of stratification derive from what has been said above:

- limitation of the risk of non-comparability;
- broader and more heterogeneous and therefore easier recruitment;
- broader representativity with a greater generalization of results;

• more sensitive statistical comparison, since the variability within each stratum is reduced when compared to the patient population as a whole;

• it offers the possibility of studying not only the effects of the treatments compared, but also the influence of prognostic factors and their interactions (potentiation, neutralization).

2.5. Drawbacks of stratification

• The most serious drawback of stratification is the limited number of strata that can be used, that is the number of independent factors that can be studied.

For example, if we wished to stratify for the "age" factor, say by decades from 20 to 60 years (i.e. 4 age-groups) and for sex (2 groups) the patient sample would be divided into 4 x 2 = 8 subgroups. If, in addition, we wished to take account of a simple index of disease severity (say 3 different degrees: mild, moderate and severe) this would make 4 x 2 x 3 = 24 subgroups.

If only two treatments were being compared, randomization would further divide these 24 subgroups into 48 subgroups. If the number of patients to be included in the trial was set at 40, it would be impossible to include patients in each subgroup. Furthermore, if some strata contain only one patient then all the benefit of stratification is lost since a single patient can obviously not be "subdivided".

If a given stratum contains three patients (in a trial comparing two treatments) randomization will necessarily attribute one of the treatments to *one* patient and the other treatment to *two* patients, thus producing an unbalanced 2/1 ratio.

The efficacy of stratification therefore diminishes if certain "cells" contain few or no patients.

Consideration of variables with little importance can be harmful to the proper balance of the essential variable.

In practice, it is seldom advisable to stratify for more than one or two factors, particularly if the anticipated total number of trial participants is relatively small.

The choice of stratification factors will thus have to be based on surveys, previous studies or on a *pilot trial* (small preliminary study of feasibility) to choose these factors. For complex subdivisions with combinations of individual categories, the ideal situation would be to have *pre-established stratification for which prognostic relevance and reproducibility have already been tested before the trial*.

• In some cases, the break in a symetric distribution of the results may yield asymmetrical distribution within strata (20).

• Finally, there are practical problems associated with stratification related to the need for separate randomization and preparation of surplus drug batches (since the number of patients recruited in each stratum is usually not known in advance). Also, great care must be taken to ensure that proper patient allocation to treatments is correctly performed within the strata, since the handling of multiple drug batches carries a certain risk of misallocation.

3. ADAPTIVE PROCEDURES (4, 19, 27, 28, 31, 37)

Some methods permit the rules of allocation to be modified during the trial period, either to balance the prognostic factors so as to ensure group comparability, or as a function of the differences in efficacy between the treatments compared.

3.1. Balancing prognostic factors as the trial progresses

Since the efficacy of stratication is limited in the case of multiple prognostic factors, several other methods have been devised to balance allocation during patient recruitment.

• Efron's method (11) considers only a single prognostic factor which corresponds to several categories in the "treatment" and "control" groups.

• If a new patient enters a subgroup (stratum) in which the two treatments are *equally* distributed at that time, then randomization is performed so as to give each treatment a 50% chance of being assigned.

• If on the contrary, a new patient enters a subgroup in which there is an imbalance between the two treatments compared, then randomization is *unbalanced* so as to favor the smaller subgroup (for example, one subgroup may be given 2/3 chances and the other 1/3).

• Pocock and Simon's method (27) allows several prognostic factors to be taken into account simultaneously.

Each new patient may be allocated to either of the treatments. For each of these possibilities, a calculation is made on what the sum of the differences in patient numbers would be (per treatment) for all the prognostic factors that concern the patient being entered.

This sum, considered as a "measure of imbalance" will be smallest for one of the treatments which is then given precedence over the others. Unbalanced randomization will give this treatment e.g. 2 out of 3 chances of being assigned and the other treatment 1 out of 3 chances.

• Freedman and White (17) described a simple method for applying this procedure manually.

• The "minimization" technique proposed by Taves (2, 8, 28, 31) does away with randomization completely. With this technique, each new patient is given the treatment for which the imbalance is smallest.
The unpredictability of treatment assignment is observed if there is a sufficiently large number of prognostic factors. (Treatment is assigned after a series of calculations that take account of the characteristics of all the patients previously entered, impossible to do in one's head).

Despite its theoretical drawback of excluding formal randomization (the random element here is the order of entry of patients with any prognostic factors), this procedure is remarkably effective for balancing the groups.

• Wei (23) proposed a method based on the *proportion* of patients exhibiting each of the characteristics considered (rather than their *number*) thus giving priority to balancing categories containing the smallest number of patients.

• Finally, Nordle and Brantmark's method permits balancing of several characteristics in a predetermined order of priority (26).

3.2. Procedures that take account of differences in efficacy between the treatments compared

Various methods have been devised to maximize the number of patients receiving the most effective of the compared treatments. These methods present an ethical advantage (21).

Such methods can be used only under rare conditions:

- the result of treatment must be assessable on a qualitative "all or none" basis (e.g. success or failure);

- the final result of treatment for a given patient must be known before treatment can be assigned to the following patient. This means that the duration of treatment must be short with regard to the interval between patient admissions;

- it must be assumed that patients entering a trial at different time points are comparable (7);

- results are generally analyzed by methods such as sequential, decisional or Bayesian, which will be discussed in chapter 14.

• The "play the winner" technique for two treatments (35) consists in assigning the same treatment to each new patient as long as it gives successes and then switching to the other treatment as soon as one patient fails.

• Robbins' (29) or Isbell's methods (23) take account of several of the earlier treatment results rather than just the last one.

• Flehinger and Louis' method (16) consists of performing unbalanced randomization in favor of the treatment that has given the best results if the groups are of comparable size, or in favor of the "least assigned treatment up to date", if the groups are markedly dissimilar in size.

• Continuous adaptation of the chances of assignment of a treatment as a function of intermediate results (34) has also been proposed.

References

1 Alderson M. Randomization. Br Med J 1975; *3*: 489.

2 Armitage P, Gehan EA. Statistical methods for the identification and use of prognostic factors. Int J Cancer 1974; *13*: 16-36.

3 Byar DP. Why data bases should not replace randomized clinical trials? Biometrics 1980; *36*: 337-42.

4 Byar DP, Simon RMD, Friedewald WT et al. Randomized clinical trials. Perspectives on some recent ideas. New Engl J Med 1976; *295*: 74-9.

5 Cancer research campaign working party. Trials and tribulation thoughts on the organization of multicentre clinical studies. Br Med J 1980; *281*: 918-20.

6 Carleton RA, Sanders CA, Burack WR. Heparin administration after acute myocardial infarction. New Engl J Med 1960; *263*: 1002-5.

7 Chalmers TC. Randomization: perils and problems. New Engl J Med 1975; *292*: 1036-7.

8 Charlson ME, Feinstein AR. The auxometric dimension: a new method for using rate of growth in pronostic staging of breast cancer. J Amer Med Assoc 1974; *228*: 180-5.

9 Coronary Drug Project Research Group: the coronary drug project: design, methods and baseline results. Circulation 1973; *47*; suppl. 1: 1-50.

10 Ederer F. Practical problems in collaborative clinical trials. Am J Epidemiol 1975; *102*: 111-8.

11 Efron B. Forcing a sequential experiment to be balanced. Biometrika 1971; *58*: 403-17.

12 Feinstein AR. Clinical epidemiology, III. The clinical design of statistics in therapy. Ann Int Med 1968; *69*: 1287-312.

13 Feinstein AR. Clinical biostatistics XIV - the purposes of prognostic stratification. Clin Pharmacol Ther 1972; *13*: 285-97.

14 Feinstein AR. Clinical biostatistics XV-XVI. The process of prognostic stratification. Clin Pharmacol Ther 1972; *13*: 442-57 and 609-24.

15 Fisher RA, Yates F. Statistical tables for biological, agricultural and medical research. 6th edition. Edinburgh: Oliver and Boyd, 1963.

16 Flehinger B, Louis TA. Sequential treatment allocation in clinical trials. Biometrika 1971; *58*: 419-26.

17 Freedman LS, White SJ. On the use of Pocock and Simon's method for balancing treatment numbers over prognostic factors in the controlled clinical trial. Biometrics 1976; *32*: 691-4.

18 Hamilton M. Lectures on the methodology of clinical research. Edinburgh: Churchill Livingstone, 1974: 115.

19 Hamilton M. On the therapies of the depressive illnesses. Evaluation of treatment. Some lessons from controlled trials. Canad Psych Ass J 1966; *11*: suppl. S86-S91.

20 Hastings WK. Variance reduction and non-normality. Biometrika 1974; *61*: 143-9.

21 Hoel DG, Sobel M, Weiss GH. A survey of adaptive sampling for clinical trials. In: Perspectives in biometrics, volume I, Elashoff RM, ed. New York: Academic Press, 1975.

22 Horwitz RI, Feinstien AR. Advantages and drawbacks of the Zelen design for randomized clinical trials. J Clin Pharmacol 1980; *20*: 425-7.

23 Isbell JR. On a problem of Robbins. Ann Math Statist 1959; *30*: 606-10.

24 Krischer JP, Hurley C, Pillalamarri M et al. An automated patient registration and treatment randomization system for multicenter clinical trials. Controlled Clinical Trials 1991; *12*: 367-77.

25 Lasagna L. Clinical trials of drugs from the viewpoint of the academic investigator (a satire). Clin Pharmacol Ther 1975; *18*: 629-33.

26 Nordle O, Brantmark BO. A self-adjusting randomization plan for allocation of patients into two treatment groups. Clin Pharm Ther 1977; *22*: 825-30.

27 Pocock SJ, Simon R. Sequential treatment assignment with balancing for prognostic factors in the controlled clinical trial. Biometrics 1975; *31*: 103-15.

28 Reed JV, Wickham EA. Practical experience of minimisation in clinical trials. Pharmaceut Med 1988; *3*: 349-59.

29 Robbins H. A sequential decision problem with a finite memory. Proc Nat Acad Sci. USA 1956; *42*: 920-3.

30 Royall RM. Current advances in sampling theory: implications for human observational studies. Amer J Epidemiol 1976; *104*: 463-74.

31 Taves DR. Minimization: a new method of assigning patients to treatment and control groups. Clin Pharmacol Ther 1974; *15*: 443-53.

32 Tiplady B. A basic program for constructing a dispensing list for a randomized clinical trial. Br J Clin Pharmacol 1981; *11*: 617-8.

33 Wei LJ. An application of an urn model to the design of sequential controlled clinical trials. J Amer Statist Assoc 1978; *73*: 559-63.

34 Weinstein MC. Allocation of subjects in medical experiments. New Engl J Med 1974; *291*: 1278-85.

35 Zelen M. Play the winner rule and the controlled clinical trial. J Am Statist Assoc 1969; *64*: 131-46.

36 Zelen M. A new desing for randomized clinical trials. New Engl J Med 1979; *300*: 1242-45.

37 Zielhuis GA, Staatman H, Van 'T Hof-Grootenboer AE, Van Lier HJJ, Rach GH, Van Den Broek P. The choice of a balanced allocation method for a clinical trial in otitis media with effusion. Statistics in Medicine 1990; *9*: 237-46.

6 - Single-blind and double-blind trials

SUMMARY

The purpose of blind trial techniques is to reduce observer bias (subjective interpretation of results and heterosuggestion) and patient bias (subjective interpretation of symptoms and autosuggestion) by concealing the identity of the treatment administered, either from the patient, the investigator, or from both.

The double-blind trial requires the following conditions:
- the drugs compared should be indistinguishable;
- the code should be accessible in case of an emergency;
- strict precautions should be taken to avoid leaks.

Sometimes, an "open" (non-blind) study may provide for "blind" interpretation of results by a third person who has contacts with neither investigator nor patients.
It is preferable to conduct an open trial rather than a false double-blind trial in which the treatments have been made blatantly obvious by "leaks" or by their characteristic effects.

One of the major concerns in designing a trial is to avoid bias, that is systematic errors that may favor one of the treatments to the detriment of the other. One of the important ways of introducing bias is to have a preconceived idea about the result. When this occurs, the investigator is always influenced in his judgment to a greater or a lesser degree, consciously or subconsciously. He can never be completely objective, nor can the patient be insensitive to the hope and confidence he places in a new treatment. Such factors may be more decisive in producing improvement than the *specific effect* of the drug (6).

If the trial is designed in such a way that either the physician or the patient does not know which treatment is being administered until the final analysis of the results, then we are performing a "single-blind" trial. If both the physician and the patient are unaware of which treatment is being given, then we are performing a "double-blind trial".

1. JUSTIFICATION FOR BLIND TRIALS (FIGURE 1)

1.1. *An investigator cannot be completely objective* in his comparison of two or more treatments. Some degree of scepticism or prejudice is inevitable and will necessarily influence his judgment. Even if he is totally impartial at the outset, the *early results* of a new drug, too preliminary to enable a conclusion to be reached, will always create some degree of enthusiasm or disappointment which it is difficult to ignore completely. Not only will this have a bearing on the results (it may introduce a "subjective" component into even the more "objective" criteria), but it may also affect motivation and recruitment for the study. If a comparative study is open (i.e. non-blind), one of the treatments is very often preferred to the other, though the preferred treatment may not necessarily be the same at the beginning and at the end of the trial.

Errors in measurement and interpretation tend more often to favor the treatment preferred. Thus, double-blind studies are generally less favorable to new treatments than open trials.

Figure 1
Bias in favor of the a priori preferred treatment

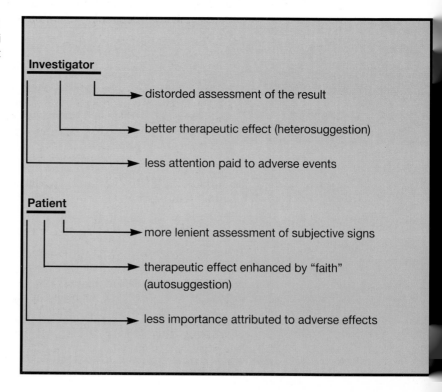

Investigator
- distorded assessment of the result
- better therapeutic effect (heterosuggestion)
- less attention paid to adverse events

Patient
- more lenient assessment of subjective signs
- therapeutic effect enhanced by "faith" (autosuggestion)
- less importance attributed to adverse effects

Finally, the enthusiasm of the physician *influences the outcome of treatment*. A treatment will be all the more effective if the prescribing physician and those responsible for patient care firmly believe in its worth use (heterosuggestion and psychotherapeutic effect). Conversely, pessimism or the physician's more or less conscious desire not to demonstrate a difference will make the comparison less sensitive.

1.2. *If the patient believes in the therapeutic value* of the treatment he is receiving, he will be favorably influenced. Not only will he tend to be more *"lenient" in interpreting* subjective improvement or in his complaints of adverse events, but also he will *actually improve* and will be less affected by the adverse events, simply as a result of autosuggestion. Of course, this improvement is not a bad thing, but it is important in a trial for patients to stand *an equal chance* of improvement and to eliminate any source of bias favoring one of the treatments compared.

1.3. Finally, regardless of investigator honesty, an "open" trial is often judged as less credible than a "blind" trial, since there is suspicion of not respecting randomization. Acceptance for publication might be jeopardized....

2. BLIND TRIAL TECHNIQUES

2.1. Single-blind trials

Single-blind trials eliminate only one of the sources of bias. The situation is very different depending on whether it is the patient or the physician who is "blind".

2.1.1. Only the patient is "blind"

If the patient is "blind", he receives an anonymous treatment, which ideally should be indistinguishable from the other treatment or treatments compared except for its therapeutic efficacy. The investigator knows which treatment the patient is receiving and he interprets its efficacy and toxicity accordingly.

This procedure requires the preparation of indistinguishable drug formulations and is rarely very useful since it entails all the constraints of a double-blind study but offers none of its advantages.

2.1.2. Only the investigator is "blind"

If it is the investigator rather than the patient who is "blind", the treatments compared need not be perfectly identical (and often cannot be made so for material reasons).

Assignment of treatment should be done blindly using the procedures described in the preceding chapter (telephone, computerized information system), avoiding the traditional game of "envelopes for treatment assignment" which involve the risk of early opening before definitive inclusion of the case is decided.

This procedure requires *two observers*: the first is the "non-blind" prescriber who instructs the patient on how to take the drug (administration modalities may differ for different drugs). During treatment, the prescribing physician records the patient's comments on how he took the drug and his complaints relating to toxicity. The second is a "blind" observer who records the data necessary for evaluating the therapeutic efficacy. The practical difficulties that such a procedure entails are obvious, as is *the risk of leaks*: even if the patient is forewarned (?), he may involuntarily divulge vital information to the "blind" observer enabling the latter to identify the treatment prescribed!

Nevertheless, this procedure has been used in clinical trials for which the drugs used could not, for technical reasons, be administered via the same route or be made to appear identical (10).

In practice, in such cases the non-blind randomized trial is preferable.

2.2. Double-blind trials

In a double-blind trial, neither the patient nor any member of the medical staff is aware of which treatment is being administered until the end of the trial.

In practice, it is not recommended to use the services of a "non-blind" third person (7) to dispense drugs of identical appearance, taken from a stock of each drug using a predetermined list. The problem with this procedure is that it requires absolute secrecy on the part of the third person and there is no guarantee against "leaks".

An even less advisable technique consists in providing the medical staff with a list indicating by a code letter (A, B) which treatment is to be administered in order of patient entry. If the prescribing physician is provided with vials labelled A and B which appear to be identical certainly a double-blind trial could be conducted but for which the two groups (A and B) are known. If for any reason, treatment "A" of a single patient is identified, then we immediately know which treatment all the other patients are receiving.

The correct method consists in preparing in advance *individual numbered packages of drugs* using a preestablished list (not available to anyone until results are analyzed) and in assigning them in order of patient entry into the trial. As an added precaution, *each numbered vial containing one of the drugs compared* may bear a tear-off label which can be attached to the patient's case report form.

The term triple-blind is sometimes used to refer to a trial analyzed by a statistician who knows the compositions of groups of patients *but not of* treatments so long as the analysis has not been completed.

2.3. How can drugs of different appearance be used in a double-blind trial?

A placebo can generally be made to resemble an active drug. Two or more active drugs being compared may, however, differ in their appearance, route and schedule of administration.

It is generally not advisable to alter the pharmaceutical formulation of a drug to make it resemble another, for example, to crush tablets and place the powder in capsules, as this may have undetermined effects on bioavailability. Placing whole or broken tablets, depending on if they are scored, directly in capsules would be more acceptable. In this case, an *in vitro* dissolution study must confirm the small incidence of this *masking* (2, 15). Reformulation of a drug requires demonstration of bioequivalence.

The double-dummy technique discussed in the following chapter has the disadvantage of increasing the number of drug units the patient must take. It also means obtaining a placebo for each of the drugs compared and therefore requires the cooperation of the drug manufacturers involved (3). Interspersion of placebo administration with that of active drug administration will "fill the gaps" if two drugs compared are given according to a different schedule (for example, single daily dose versus several daily doses)*. In this case it must be ensured that the drug is packaged so that there can be no confusion between which dose should be taken at which time.

In many cases, there is no truly practical and satisfactory solution, particularly for long-term treatments, and one must then resort to a single-blind or a non-blind randomized design or choose another control drug.

2.4. Disclosing the identity of the treatment. When and how?

The pre-established list used to prepare drug packages for each patient must of course be made inaccessible to the medical staff and to the investigator's team involved with the protocol. At the end of the trial, this list will serve to break the treatment code. This decoding operation should be performed as late as possible, after all the data from the last patient has been collected and after all the data has been thoroughly checked. In practice, only the department responsible for the preparation of the drugs during the labelling phase is in possession of the list of correspondence between patient numbers and the nature of the treatment. This list is then immediately placed in a secret and inaccessible location except for a documented "break-in". It is only after correction and validation of all data in the trial (data freezing) that the statistician obtains access to the correspondence list.

* But the profit of "once daily dose" concerning adherence to treatment is lost.

2.5. Procedures for emergency situations

In case of an emergency, such as the need for general anesthesia or an attempted suicide, accidental ingestion of the drug by a small child, etc. it may be necessary to break the code for an individual patient. For this purpose, a series of numbered envelopes should be prepared in advance to enable immediate identification of the treatment administered to any given patient. Thus, breaking the code for one patient will not disclose the treatments of the other patients. It is wise to make sure that the envelopes cannot be easily steam-opened and closed again and that the contents cannot easily be read by transillumination (even with a halogen lamp). Avoiding this type of indiscretion is difficult indeed, especially if the envelopes are accessible to several members of the medical staff. It thus is important that all envelopes opened immediately be dated and signed and to inform all those involved with the protocol that all the envelopes will be *recovered and checked* at the end of the trial.

A computer can be used to automatically prepare one or several series of tamperproof opaque envelopes, on the outside of which only the patient's identification number appears, the treatment code being placed on the inside. This automated procedure prevents errors made by hand.

Another procedure consists in using miniature envelopes attached to the label of the drug vial (flag envelopes). This envelope is detached from the label as each vial is attributed to a patient and it can then be attached to the case report form (4).

Another technique is to use sheets of thin cardboard with multiple, small detachable "windows" each allowing the code to be broken for one patient at a time (principle of the "Advent calendar").

Finally, some poison control centers accept to keep a series of decoding envelopes in case of an emergency (and if the trial involves a new drug, an information file on it). If the trial is conducted in a hospital, it is also possible to give the envelopes and the relevant documentation to the hospital pharmacist. All envelopes are recovered and checked at the end of the trial.

2.6. "Blind" reading or interpretation of results

When single or double-blind methods are impractical, and if the criterion of response can be evaluated by a biological specimen or a permanent record (X-ray film, tracing), the result can be read "blind". To do this, the specimen, film, or tracing is submitted to an assessor independent of the medical staff and the assays, evaluations or measurement are made without any interference from the latter until the final analysis of the data.

2.7. Blind time

A still more elaborate procedure, proposed for the study of psychotropic drugs, consists in questioning the subject in front of a television camera and recording the interview on video tape (4, 13, 14). This *"blind time"* procedure makes it possible to present successive interviews to the observer in random order. Thus, he is not influenced from one test to another by knowing the results of the preceding tests. This procedure requires the erasing of passages on the tape during which the patient gives information enabling the identification of the time and the treatment.

In pharmacokinetics, it can be useful to make assays in coded tubes for which the chronological order of sample collection is not known to avoid subconsiously smoothing out of curves.

3. FALSE DOUBLE-BLIND TRIALS

The possibility of leaks, discussed earlier, carres a risk of completely distorting the results of the trial, which, being no longer blind, loses all the advantages of this method while retaining only its practical constraints (18).

Consequently, no effort should be spared to ensure that the code is hidden, that the envelopes are tamperproof (*or that any attempt to cheat can readily be detected*) and that the drugs compared really are indistinguishible. Indeed, sometimes the medical staff attaches greater importance to the "guess who got what" game (sometimes to alleviate latent anxiety due to their uncertainty) than to the unbiased comparison of drug effects.

When the subjects in the trial partake in such "games", then there is no limit to the potential sources of error. During a trial a patient may bring his drug to a pharmacist to be analyzed (this actually happened!). The National Institutes of Health (NIH) in the USA designed a trial (12) to compare vitamin C with a placebo in volunteers recruited ... among NIH personnel! Some of the participants lost no time in opening capsules and tasting the contents to identify the preparation they were receiving and many succeeded. The results of this trial were probably at least partly distorted by this behavior: the authors who published the results admitted the fact with total (and unusual) frankness. It is quite conceivable that in other instances, similar errors were overlooked or concealed! In the Aspirin Myocardial Infarction Study (A.M.I.S.), a post hoc investigation revealed that many patients tried to guess the nature of the treatment and often succeeded in doing so ... (9).

In some cases, the nature of a treatment may be revealed to the clinician by its therapeutic or adverse effects. Surprisingly, even the most alert clinicians often err in this venture. For example, a change in heart rate "should" theoretically make it possible to distinguish a beta-blocker from a placebo. But in practice, the ranges of heart rates in both treatment groups overlap so widely that it is impossible for a specific subject to identify the treatment *with certainty* (17). If it is known that this is the case, then one can pass over this risk of identification, unless an obvious effect reveals one of the treatments with virtual certainty after it is administered (e.g. laboratory testing of hemostasis in treatment with an anticoagulant).

Thus, the resemblance between a placebo and an active drug must be as perfect as possible from the standpoint of color, shape, appearance and dimensions. It is better not to try to simulate the taste and smell, unless these are due to the presence of the excipients, under penalty of introducing substances whose possible therapeutic action has not been tested... It is recommended to submit the placebo and the active drug to an *ad hoc* committee to assess resemblance by systematically looking for differences (1, 5, 8, 16).

If a double-blind trial thus proves impossible to conduct, it is preferable to run an open but correctly done comparative study (11).

Regardless of the source of the unwanted decoding, it is always more serious when it occurs before selection of patients rather than during the course of treatment, because, in addition to a bias in evaluation, it results in a selection bias.

4. LIMITS OF BLIND METHODS

Aside from the case of a false double-blind study discussed above, other difficulties occur. For example, if one of the treatments compared consists of a drug which requires *dosage adjustment* according to the patient's response, it will often be difficult to perform a double-blind trial, though it remains possible. Placebo doses can be "adjusted", or a second non-blind observer can adjust doses. For example, a coordinating center can, in view of the results of a laboratory test, decide to increase the dosage for a patient under treatment with the active drug, and simultaneously to maintain the double-blind, decide to increase the dose given to a patient on placebo.

If *long-term treatment is planned* (for several months or even years), the problem of maintenance (distribution of the same anonymous drug to the same patient) and especially the increasing risk of leaks makes the success of a double-blind trial more chancy.

In all cases, it is often possible to perform a single-blind or even a non-blind study. Such studies are always preferable to a hypocritical or naively false double-blind trial in which the code is in fact no more than an open secret!

References

1 Anderson TW, Ashley MJ, Clarke EA. Not so double-blind? Br Med J 1976; *1*: 457-8.

2 Bernstein DF, Tiano FJ. Preparation, packaging and labeling of investigational drug supplies. Part I: preparation of investigational drug supplies. J Clin Res Pharmacoepidemiol 1991; *5*: 1-10.

3 Berry H. Drug firm's cooperation in clinical trials. Br Med J 1978; *2*: 497.

4 Bronstein J. An efficient labelling system speeds drugs to the clinic. Drug Information Journal 1981; *15*: 25-8.

5 Dupin-Spriet T, Spriet A. Circuit du médicament. Bonnes pratiques de fabrication, bonnes pratiques cliniques. Thérapie 1990; *46*: 69-74.

6 Ederer F. Patient bias, investigator bias, and the double-masked procedure in clinical trials. Amer J Med 1975; *58*: 295-9.

7 Heller A, Zahourek R, Whittington MG. Effectiveness of anti-depressant drugs: a triple-blind study comparing imipramine, desimipramine and placebo. Amer J Pysychiat 1971; *127*: 1092-5.

8 Hill LE, Nunn AJ, Fox W. Matching quality of agents employed in a "double-blind" controlled clinical trial. Lancet 1976; *1*: 352-6.

9 Howard J, Wittemore AS, Hoover JJ et al. How blind was the patient blind in AMIS? Clin Pharmacol Ther 1982; *32*: 543-53.

10 Huskisson EC, Gibson TJ, Balme HW et al. Trial comparing d-penicillamine and gold in rheumatoid arthritis. Ann Rheum Dis 1974; *33*: 532-5.

11 Huskisson EC, Scott J. How double blind is double-blind? and does it matter? Br J Clin Pharm 1976; *3*: 331-2.

12 Karlowski TR, Chalmers TC, Frenkel LD, Zapikian AZ, Lewis TL, Lynch JM. Ascorbic acid for the common cold: a prophylactic and therapeutic trial. J Amer Med Assoc 1975; *231*: 1038-42.

13 Mormont C, Von Frenckell R, Lottin T, Mormont I, Troisfontaines B, Bobon D. Influences de variables temporelles (time-blind, time gap) sur l'évaluation quantitative de la psychopathologie. L'Encéphale 1984; *10*: 3-7.

14 Renfordt E, Busch H. Time-blind analysis of TV-scored interviews. An objective method to study antidepressive drug-effects. Pharmacopsychiat 1976; *11*: 129-34.

15 Spriet A, Dupin-Spriet T. a) Bonne pratique des essais cliniques des médicaments. Bâle: Karger, 1990. b) Good practice of clinical drug trials. Basel: Karger, 1992.

16 Vere DW, Chaput de Saintonge DM. Double-blind trials. Lancet 1976; *i*: 546.

17 Yorkston NY, Gruzelier JH, Zaki SA, Hollander D, Pitcher DR, Sergeant HGS. Propranolol in chronic schizophrenia. Lancet 1977; *ii*: 1082-3.

18 Zifferblatt SM, Wilbur CS. A psychological perspective for double blind trials. Clin Pharmacol Ther 1978; *23*: 1-10.

7 - Choice of the comparator: placebo or active drug?

SUMMARY

A controlled trial of a treatment is conducted in comparison to a placebo or an active control treatment. This choice is made taking into account many considerations, and keeping in mind that the smaller the difference in therapeutic efficacy, the more difficult it is to demonstrate. The simultaneous comparison of a new treatment with a placebo and an active control validates the comparison if the latter is proven to be more effective than the placebo.

Independent of the actual pharmacological effect of a drug, its efficacy depends on a number of non-specific factors responsible for what is globally termed the placebo effect.

To identify the pharmacological effect of a compound, it may be justifiable to compare a supposedly active drug with a placebo, a "pseudo-drug" identical in appearance but pharmacologically inert.

Factors underlying the placebo effect include the subject's personality (placebo responder or non-responder), the conditions of administration and the appearance of the drug.

The placebo effect does not appear to present distinctive characteristics which distinguish it from a true pharmacological effect and it may even be associated with adverse effects (nocebo effect).

A placebo may be used to demonstrate the efficacy of a pharmacologically active preparation but also to validate comparisons between active drugs, to facilitate the resemblance of two active drugs (double-dummy technique), to establish the relevance of different dosages or schedules of administration, to compare drug combinations with their individual components, or finally, during wash-out periods.

Selecting placebo non-responders is sometimes specified to make the comparison more sensitive.

So-called "impure placebos" (i.e. drugs of dubious efficacy or preparations producing the same side-effects as the active drug under study) should be avoided since the results may subsequently prove impossible to interpret.

The choice of a standard drug takes account of medical, regulatory, pharmaceutical and economic criteria.

The condition of a patient after a period of treatment depends on several criteria. It is sometimes difficult to estimate the role of each one: natural history of the disease (15), true pharmacological effect, "non specific" factors (29, 30) due to the fact that the patient is being looked after and that he believes to be receiving an active treatment. It is the latter effect which constitutes the *placebo* effect when it results in a therapeutic effect, but when it is manifested by undesirable effects it is termed a *nocebo effect* (17, 27).

The importance of the placebo effect often justifies the use of a *"placebo"*, which may be defined as a *pharmacologically inert pseudo-drug* identical in appearance to the active drug to which it is compared.

In the context of clinical trials, an active control refers to a medication whose efficacy has been proven previously, for the indication under study.

1. WHICH TREATMENTS ARE TO BE COMPARED?

The first question that needs to be asked is: should the treatment in question be compared to a placebo or to an active control?

The answer depends on the hypothesis tested and ethical limitations. Generally speaking, in a placebo-controlled comparison, the chances of finding a statistically-significant and clinically-valuable result are higher if two drugs assumed to be active are compared, even if they differ in efficacy.

• Comparison between the placebo and the active drug is intended to prove the *intrinsic pharmacological action* of the drug tested.

• Comparison with an active drug is intended to demonstrate any difference in activity (but the smaller this difference, the more difficult it is to demonstrate).

When a comparison with an active control is undertaken, it is rare that a new drug is thought to have a markedly better efficacy (and thus easy to demonstrate) (22). This is why most commonly one is led to demonstrate only the lack of a notable difference, i.e. "equivalence within Δ" (41), as discussed in chapter 2.

The difference sought, Δ must then be smaller than in a placebo-controlled trial. Otherwise, this would lead to think that two treatments are equivalent, whose difference might be as large as that which exists between the active drug and the placebo, (which would be absurd).

A well-designed trial in comparison to an active control thus requires many more cases than one versus a placebo. This is even more accentuated by the need for a two-tailed statistical test between two drugs assumed to be active while often a one-tailed test can be run to analyze the results obtained versus a placebo. All of these items of comparison are presented in table I.

Table 1
Items involved in choosing the comparator

	Placebo	Active control
Objective	Real pharmacological effect	At least : "equivalence" with a proven treatment And, if possible, improvement in comparison to an older treatment
Difference sought Δ	Large	Small
Analysis	One-tailed possibly	Two-tailed test always + Confidence interval (equivalence)
Number of cases	Small	Large
Major problem	Ethical considerations (selection of cases)	Choice of a "recognized" drug and Equitable conditions of administration

In addition, if a new drug has only been compared to an active control (without a placebo-controlled trial), this is not a convincing proof of efficacy (even if equivalence can be demonstrated).

Eligibility criteria and trial conditions have perhaps determined the improvement (or lack of improvement) in all patients, regardless of the treatment received.

This is why, in practice, the logical development of a drug generally leads first to demonstrate its efficacy in at least one or two placebo-controlled trials before undertaking comparisons with an active drug. Of course, there are exceptions, in particular in the field of oncology.

Sometimes, it is decided to simultaneously compare in the same trial the new drug to the placebo and to an active control. If the latter proves its superiority over the placebo, the sensitivity of the trial is validated. But the lack of statistical significance is not enough if equivalence, with an acceptable margin of error, is not demonstrated.

The theoretical possibility of an active drug (?), supposed to improve the disorder but actually making it worse should be kept in mind. In this case an inactive agent, by contrast, will be found to be effective.

Finally, an ethical paradox may be noted. A placebo-controlled trial appears a priori to be more harmful for the subjects in a trial than one with an active drug. Nonetheless, given the fact that it requires many fewer cases, the number of patients treated with an inactive product is lower when the drug under study is not effective. This is true for many compounds which need not then pass on to the next phase of investigation.

2. THE USE OF PLACEBOS

2.1. Non-specific effects and the placebo effect

"Non-specific" effects (figure 1) are operative *even if the product administered has no actual pharmacodynamic properties*. They can be explained by the effects of packaging, the patient's beliefs and expectations (autosuggestion) and the physician's enthusiasm (heterosuggestion) and the very fact that the subjects are participating in a trial and that they are being cared for (15, 18, 29, 30).

These non-specific factors include the influence of the patient's personality, the environment, the route of administration, and the drug that the subject believes to be (or at least can be) effective. It is the latter aspect which defines the placebo effect strictly speaking.

Figure 1
Factors influencing the effect

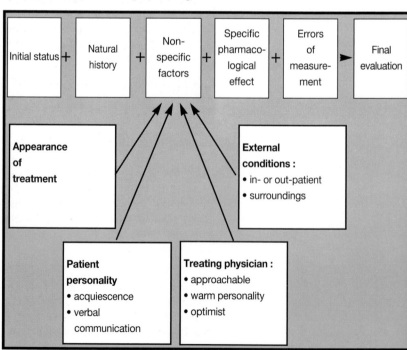

2.1.1. Placebo responders and non-responders

Some subjects respond more readily to the administration of placebos than others. Many studies have focused on the respective characteristics of these patients in the hope of defining a typical profile for the "placebo responder" and the "placebo non-responder".

No convincing correlations have been demonstrated between placebo responsiveness and physiological or demographic characteristics (20, 26, 36).

Certainly if many statistical comparisons are carried out in an effort to detect such a relationship, some patient characteristics will appear related to placebo-sensitivity. But the statistical interpretation of many tests in the same subjects is risky and requires independent confirmation. For example, the relationship found by Moertel (26) between non-smokers, educational level, occupation, marital status and number of children, on the one hand, and placebo-responsiveness, on the other hand, requires confirmation. Lasagna (20) found a relationship between sex, intelligence and response to placebos.

The study of the subject's psychological profile has proved to be particularly interesting. Patient *acquiescence* (25, 27, 28) evaluated by appropriate rating scales, appears to be related to placebo responsiveness (and thus to smaller differences in efficacy between placebo and active treatment). Similarly, a "general variability" scale (38) might also be useful in identifying placebo-responders. Finally, intelligence as assessed by verbal ability may affect the outcome of placebo treatment, at least in neurotic patients (31).

An important factor in the patient's history is the *duration of illness* and *previous medications* received (32). Patients with long-standing disease who have received more previous treatments tend to be poorer placebo responders (and hence the placebo-active treatment difference would tend to be greater).

It is probable, however, that patients who respond to a placebo for a given illness, will not necessarily have the same profile as the placebo responders for another illness or under different conditions. Also, it should be remembered that most studies on placebo response have been performed with psychotropic drugs.

Finally, the disorder treated is also an important factor in determining the extent of the placebo effect observed. A placebo effect can be achieved in a wide variety of disorders (4, 18), but the less serious the illness and the weaker the actual pharmacological effect of the treatment, the more important the role assumed by the placebo effect (14).

2.1.2. Influence of the medical staff

The efficacy of a treatment depends very much on the attitude of those responsible for patient care and particularly on the "doctor-patient" relationship. Optimistic or enthusiastic investigators achieve better results than the pessimistic or sceptical ones (3, 25, 45).

An investigator who manifests an "experimental" attitude will be less effective than a physician who adopts a "therapeutic" attitude (29); patients who consider their doctor to be "warm" (understanding) generally show better improvement than those who qualify their doctor as "cold" (indifferent) (34).

Finally, different instructions given to patients about the same treatment may have a notable influence on the outcome of the treatment (23).

2.1.3. Influence of external factors

The patient's environment may also have an influence on the outcome of treatment. For certain illnesses in particular, the placebo-active treatment difference may be very different for inpatients and outpatients (6, 33). Similarly, this result may also be influenced by the patient's family and friends (and by other patients in the hospital!).

2.1.4. Influence of the drug's appearance

The influence of the drug's appearance on its therapeutic effect can be studied by administering the same drug presented differently (assuming different identical bioavailability).

Trials based on this principle, comparing tablets and capsules of various shapes and colors, have not yet yielded unequivocal results (16, 35, 37).

The route of administration might play a more important role, particularly if injections or intravenous infusions are used, as well as the name given to the drug (5).

2.2. Characteristics of the placebo effect (2, 19, 40)

The placebo effect has been compared to the "true" pharmacological effect. It has been claimed that the former can be recognized through a number of distinctive characteristics: short duration, diminishing effect on repeated doses, and no adverse effects. In fact, the only difference between the effect of an active treatment (if it really is effective) and the placebo effect might be a difference in the degree of the effects.

In some circumstances, the duration of the placebo effect has been shown to be as long as that of the active treatment and also to be cumulative (21). With regard to the "fading-out" of the placebo effect after repeated doses, the same effect can be observed with many active drugs. Repeated doses of either placebo or active treatment have been observed to produce *increasingly better results* (26).

As for adverse effects, they are commonly observed in patients on placebos and are referred to as the nocebo reaction (10, 17). The incidence of the nocebo reaction is probably influenced by personality traits (11). "Contagion" between patients who discuss their treatment with each other, may account for the fact that in a clinical trial the patients receiving the placebo often complain of the *same* adverse effects as patients receiving the active drug (8).

2.3. Various methods of using placebos

A placebo may be used in a therapeutic trial to compare its effects with those of the active drug, but also to validate a comparison between two supposedly active drugs, to allow "blind" administration of two drugs that cannot be made indistinguishible (double-dummy technique), to study drug combinations, and to permit therapeutic withdrawal periods.

2.3.1. The simple "placebo versus active drug" trial

This simple design makes it possible to distinguish the actual pharmacological effect of an assumedly active drug. Of course, the absence of a significant difference between a placebo and an active medication does not necessarily mean that the latter is ineffective. The criterion chosen may not have been sensitive enough or there may not have been enough patients in the trial.

The placebo concept may be extended to areas other than those of drugs:

• in surgery, a sham operation may be performed consisting of anesthesia and incision of the skin (3, 7);

• in dietetics, foods (39) or even complete diets (9) that look alike but differ in their composition can be used;

• "placebo points" can be used in acupuncture (12, 44);

• in electroconvulsive therapy, the procedure can be limited to positioning the electrodes and anesthesia (43).

2.3.2. Comparison of active drugs validated by a placebo

If the comparison of a new drug A with a proven drug B shows no significant difference, there is no way of knowing whether the absence of difference is not due to an insufficiently sensitive method of evaluating the results under the conditions of the trial.

Adding a placebo makes the trial a three-way comparison (drug A, drug B, placebo) and eliminates the possibility of insufficient sensitivity if the proven drug turns out to be superior to the placebo. This procedure is sometimes referred to as the comparison of a drug with a "positive" control and with a "negative" control, i.e. the placebo.

This procedure may be useful in trials involving new drugs but it is occasionally difficult to interpret, as for example, when the "best" and "worst" treatments are significantly different, whereas the "intermediate" treatment does not differ significantly from either.

2.3.3. The double-dummy technique

If two drugs A and B cannot be made to look exactly alike, it is nevertheless possible to compare them in a double-blind manner by giving A with a placebo of B, and B with a placebo of A. Each patient thus is given two drugs simultaneously, an active drug and a placebo, and the two treatments are indistinguishable.

The same approach can be used for comparing two drugs that must be administered by different routes, for example, an injectable preparation and an oral drug. This necessarily implies giving injections of a placebo together with an active preparation administered orally, and may raise objections from the ethical standpoint.

Finally the double-dummy technique can be used when different schedules are required for two drugs administered via the same route but with different times of administration.

The problem with the double-dummy method is that it increases the number of drug doses the patient has to take. Thus in a trial comparing two drugs in dissimilar tablet form, the use of the double-dummy technique meant that each patient had to take 16 tablets a day (24).

2.3.4. Comparison of a drug combination with each of its components

If it is wished to compare the effects of a drug combination A + B with those of each of its components administered alone, patients receiving A can be given a placebo resembling B and vice-versa.

The trial thus can be conducted "double-blind" and each patient receives the same number of daily doses. It is better to add a fourth group receiving the two placebos according to a factorial design (figure 2):

Figure 2
Factorial design to study drug combinations

A + B	B + Placebo (A)
A + Placebo (B)	Placebo (A) + Placebo (B)

2.3.5. Withdrawal period

When prior treatment has to be discontinued at the start of a trial or between two phases of a trial, there must be a withdrawal or "wash-out" period. If it is undesirable to leave patients without any form of treatment a placebo that resembles the drugs compared may be administered, but this can hardly be done "double-blind". *The withdrawal period cannot therefore, be considered unreservedly as a "control period" to compare the assumedly active drugs with the placebo.* The withdrawal period can, however, be used for studying the patients' baseline status, their stability and group comparability.

2.4. Problems raised by the use of placebos

Several problems associated with the use of placebos warrant consideration: selection of placebo non-responders, imperfect likeness, "impure" placebos and ethical problems.

2.4.1. Exclusion of placebo responders or active drug non-responders (13)

In placebo responders, the likelihood of observing a difference between the drug studied and the placebo is less than in placebo non-responders. It is therefore tempting to make an effort to restrict patient selection to the latter group with a view to making the comparison more sensitive. In theory, two methods may be used for this purpose:

• Subjects who exhibit a "placebo reactor profile" may be excluded *a priori*. However, subjects who respond to a placebo for a given type of treatment or disorder may not necessarily do so for others. The procedure used for designating placebo reactors should therefore have been validated for the *trial undertaken*. Furthermore, the subjects more resistant to a placebo response are often also the most "treatment-resistant" and hence there is little to be gained in terms of the active treatment-placebo *difference*.

• The second method is a decision of *a posteriori* selection, following a *pre-trial phase prior to the randomized period* during which all potential participants are given the placebo. Those patients who respond "too well" are excluded.

Exclusion of subjects who do not respond to the active drug according to the inverse schema involves a first non-comparative phase of administration of the active drug to all subjects. Selection for the randomized phase retains only the responders (1).

In all cases, the aim sought is sensitization of the comparison to decrease the number of patients randomized.

2.4.2. Expiry of the placebo

Except sometimes for withdrawal periods, placebos usually are used in a *"double-blind"* design. Thus, the placebo should match the active drug as closely as possible throughout the duration of its utilization. This is why it is preferable to define and check a date for expiry of the placebo which, in fact, only involves the duration of resemblance to the active drug. For example, differences in color have been observed which developed after a period of months (42).

2.4.3. Impure placebos

We may sometimes hesitate to give patients a pharmacologically inactive preparation and may prefer to give them an older drug of *doubtful efficacy* or very low doses of uncertain efficacy of an active preparation. This procedure should be avoided since it may render the comparison uninterpretable. If, for example, the results show that the new treatment is equivalent to the older treatment, the former will be classified among the category of drugs of "doubtful efficacy" which is obviously not the purpose of the trial!

When a drug under study has virtually constant and characteristic adverse effects which distinguish it clearly from the placebo, the double-blind design may be relative, although in practice mistaken recognition is frequent. To overcome this problem, the use of an "impure placebo" with the *same* effects as the active medication has been recommended. For example, atropine may be added to the placebo for an antidepressant that produces anticholinergic effects. This procedure *must be rejected* since it cannot be stated with certainty beforehand that the "impurity" added to the placebo will have no effect, either positive or negative, on the course of the disorder treated. Furthermore, it is ethically questionable to knowingly induce adverse effects in patients without any intent of therapeutic benefit.

2.4.4. Ethical safeguards

To limit the drawback of having no effective treatment for the disorder under study, the protocol can contain safeguards such as:
- voluntary early discontinuation of treatment (the percentage of patients who continue on treatment or the duration of treatment become the principal criterion of response),
- addition of a symptomatic treatment at the patient's request,
- administration of study treatments in addition to the routine basic treatment.

All these conditions do not rule out the use of a placebo during phase 4 trials which once again still becomes very useful:
- if the benefit/risk ratio for the registered drug is modified,
- if the methodology of previous studies is unsatisfactory,
- if the results of previous studies are debatable,
- if one seeks to demonstrate a long-term effect (longer duration than during phase 3 studies).

3. CHOICE OF THE STANDARD DRUG

3.1. Medical criteria

When one seeks to compare a *new* drug to a *recognized* treatment, it is important to choose the latter carefully.

Several cases are possible:

- If there is a "classical" treatment of unquestionable therapeutic value, it is desirable that it at least be used in a controlled trial as the control treatment. Aspirin can be mentioned which is commonly used as a "standard" in the study of minor analgesics.

- If, in addition, there are newer medications which have advantages in comparison to the classical standard drug, it is logical to also use them as controls. Theoretically, it appears evident that *the* treatment selected as the standard drug should be the "best known treatment". In practice, it often is not possible to propose an unquestionable hierarchy of different existing treatments that are classified according to their therapeutic value. Indeed, the evaluation of the *known* advantages and drawbacks of different drugs changes over time from one country to another; moreover, sometimes new properties are discovered for older drugs. Furthermore, if one treatment were unanimously and definitively recognized as being the best for all patients, use of the other treatments would not longer be justified...

For this reason, comparison against *several* active drugs are planned, generally in separate trials since trials with multiple treatments often pose serious problems in the interpretation of their results.

3.2. Regulatory criteria

The comparator used in a given country must, in order to be considered as a standard drug, be registered in that country for the indication, dosage and pharmaceutical formulation specified in the protocol. This makes it complicated to conduct international multicenter trials.

3.3. Pharmaceutical criteria

If one seeks to conduct a double-blind trial, the feasibility of the pharmaceutical formulation, without overly complicating the modalities for administration nor compromising compliance with therapy, often guides the choices of the comparator (17).

3.4. Economic criteria

If a new drug does not possess clear therapeutic superiority over existing treatments, it nevertheless can be more or less expensive and this factor must also be taken into consideration. It thus is important that the sponsor of the trial takes into account the costs of treatments chosen as standard drugs, a factor that is used, moreover, in some countries, by the regulatory authorities who set drug prices.

References

1 Amery W, Dony JA. Clinical trial design avoiding undue placebo treatment. J Clin Pharmacol 1975; *15*: 674-9.

2 Beecher HK. The powerful placebo. J Amer Med Assoc 1955; *155*: 1602-6.

3 Beecher HK. Surgery as placebo. A quantitative study of bias.J Amer Med Assoc 1961; *176*: 1102-7.

4 Benson H, Epstien MD. The placebo effect. A neglected aspect in the care of patients. J Amer Med Assoc 1975; *232*: 1225-7.

5 Branthwaite A, Cooper P. Analgesic effects of branding in treatment of headaches. Br Med J 1981; *282*: 1576-8.

6 Chadha DR, Dasilva LM. The placebo effects in clinical psychopharmacology. Current Therapeutic Research 1977; *21*: S 748-S 52.

7 Cobb LA, Thomas GI, Dillard DH, Merendino KA, Bruce RA. An evaluation of internal-mammary ligation by a double-blind technique. New Engl J Med 1950; *260*: 1115-8.

8 Cromie BW. The feet of clay of the double-blind trial. Lancet 1963; *2*: 994-7.

9 Dayton S, Pearce ML, Hashimoto S, Dixon WJ, Tomiyasu U. A clinical trial of a diet high in unsaturated fat in preventing complications of atherosclerosis. Circulation 1969; *40*: suppl. II 1-63.

10 Dhume VC, Agshikar NV, Diniz RS. Placebo-induced side-effects in healthy volunteers. The Clinician 1975; *39*: 289-91.

11 Downing RW, Rickels K, Meyers F. Self-report of hostility and the incidence of side-reactions in neurotic out-patients treated with tranquilizing drugs and placebo. J Consulting Psychol 1967; *31*: 71-6.

12 Gaw AC, Chang LW, Shaw LC. Efficacy of acupuncture on osteoarthritic pain. A controlled double-blind study. New Engl J Med 1975; *293*: 375-8.

13 Haegerstam G, Huitfeld B, Nilsson BS, Sjövall J, Syvälahti E, Walhén A. Placebo in clinical drug trials - a multidisciplinary review. Meth and Find Exper Clin Pharmacol 1982; *4*: 261-78.

14 Hamilton M. Discussion of the meeting. In: Rickels K, ed. Non-specific factors in drug therapy. Springfield: Charles C.Thomas, 1968: 133-35.

15 Honigfeld G. Specific and non-specific factors in the treatment of depressed states. In: Rickels K, ed. Non-specific factors in drug therapy. Springfield: Charles C. Thomas, 1968; 80-107.

16 Hussain MZ. Effect of shape of medication in treatment of anxiety states. Br J Psychiat 1972; *120*: 507-9.

17 Kennedy WP. The nocebo reaction. Med World 1961; *95*: 203-5.

18 Kissel P, Barrucand D. Placebos et effect placebo en médecine. Paris: Masson, 1964.

19 Lachaux B, Lemoine P. Placebo. Un médicament qui cherche la vérité. Paris: Medsi/McGraw Hill 1988.

20 Lasagna L, Mostellier F, Von Felsinger JM, Beecher HK. A study of the placebo response. Am J Med 1954; *16*: 770-9.

21 Lasagna L, Laties VG, Dohan JL. Further studies on the "pharmacology" of placebo administration. J Clin Invest 1958; *37*: 553-7.

22 Leber P. The placebo control in clinical trials (A view from the FDA). Psychopharmacol Bull 1986; *22*: 30-2.

23 Lyerly SB, Ross S, Krugman AD, Clyde DJ. Drugs and placebos. The effects of instructions upon performance and mood under amphetamine sulphate and chloral hydrate. J Abnormal Social Psychology 1964; *68*: 321-7.

24 McLellan DL, Chalmers RJ, Johnson RH. A double-blind trial of tetra-benazine thiopropazate and placebo in patients with chorea. Lancet 1974; *1*: 104-7.

25 McNair DM, Kahn RJ, Dropplema LF, Fisher S. Patient acquiescence and drug effects. In: Rickels K ed. Non-specific factors in drug therapy. Springfield: Charles C. Thomas, 1968: 59-72.

26 Moertel CG, Taylor WF, Roth A, Tyce FA. Who responds to sugar pills? Mayo Clinic Proc 1976; *50*: 96-100.

27 Pichot P, Perse J. Placebo effects as response set. In: Rickels K, ed. Non-specific factors in drug therapy. Springfield: Charles C. Thomas 1968: 50-8.

28 Pichot P. La nature de l'effect placebo. In: La relation médecin-malade au cours des chimiothérapies. Lambert PA, ed. Paris: Masson, 1965

29 Rickels K. Non-specific factors in drug therapy of neurotic patients. In: Non-specific factors in drug therapy. Springfield: Charles C. Thomas, 1968: 3-26.

30 Rickels K. Non-specific factors in drug treatment. In: Brady JP, Orme MT, Riegber W, ed. Psychiatry areas of promise and advancement. New York: Spectrum Press, 1976.

31 Rickels K, Downing R. Verbal ability (intelligence) and improvement in drug therapy of neurotic patients. J New Drugs 1965; *5*: 303-7.

32 Rickels K, Lipman R, Raab E. Previous medication, duration of illness, and placebo responses. J Nerv Ment Dis. 1966; *142*: 548-54.

33 Rickels K, Clark E, Etezady MH, Sachs T, Sapra RK, Yee R. Butabarbital sodium and chlordiazepoxide in anxious patients: a collaborative controlled study. Clin Pharmacol Ther 1970; *11*: 538-50.

34 Rickels R, Lipman, RS, Park LC, Covi L, Uhlenhuth EH, Mock JE. Drug, doctor warmth, and clinic setting in the symptomatic response to minor tranquilizers. Psychopharmacologia (Berl.) 1971; *20*: 128-52.

35 Schapira K, McClelland HA, Griffiths NR, Newell DJ. Study of the effects of tablet colour in the treatment of anxiety states. Br Med J 1970; *2*: 446-9.

36 Shapiro K, Struening EL, Barten H, Shapiro E. Correlates of placebo reaction in an outpatient population. Psychological Medicine 1975; *5*: 389-96.

37 Schiff AA, Murphy JE, Anderson JA. Non-pharmacological factors in drug therapy: the interaction of doctor, patient and tablet appearance in the treatment of anxiety/depression syndromes. J Int Med Res 1975; *3*: 125-33.

38 Sharp HC. Identifying placebo-reactors. J Psychol 1965; *60*: 205-12.

39 Soltoft J, Krag B, Gudmand-Hoyer E, Kristensen E, Wulff HR. A double-blind trial of the effect of wheat bran on symptoms of irritable bowel syndrome. Lancet 1965; *1*: 270-2.

40 Spiro HM. Doctors, patients and placebos. New Haven: Yale University Press, 1986.

41 Spriet A, Beiler D. When can "non-significantly different" treatments be considered as "equivalent"? Br J Clin Pharmacol 1979; *7*: 623-4.

42 Spriet A, Dupin-Spriet T. a) Bonne pratique des essais cliniques des médicaments. Bâle: Karger, 1990. b) Good practice of clinical drug trials. Basel: Karger, 1992.

43 Tetreault L, Bordeleau JM. Expérience contrôlée en psychopharmacologie clinique. In: Actualités de thérapeutiques psychiatriques. 3ème série. Paris: Masson, 1972: 9-20.

44 Weintraub M, Peturson S, Schwartz M et al. Acupuncture in musculo-skeletal pain: methodology and results in a double-blind controlled trial. Clin Pharmacol Ther 1975; *17*: 248.

45 Wheatley D. Effects of doctors' and patients' attitude and other factors on response to drugs. In: Rickels K, eds. Non-specific factors in drug therapy. Springfield: Charles C. Thomas, 1968: 73-9.

8 - Dosage and therapeutic schema

SUMMARY

In a drug development program, it is generally necessary to study the dose-response relationship by comparing several dosages of the drug. The treatments compared can be administered in fixed or variable dosage depending on the trial objective. Adjustment of doses is difficult in a double-blind trial and can sometimes be done before the patient is entered into the actual comparative trial. Studies of dosage are conducted either by trials of strict dose-response relationship (parallel groups receiving different doses) or by trials of forced or non-forced titration (dose progression in each subject until a threshold is reached).

The administration schedule should also be optimal for each drug and this may require the use of the "double-dummy" technique, where placebos are added to exactly duplicate the administration schedule.

In some cases, ancillary treatment may be considered as incompatible with the trial and the patient will have to be excluded if he cannot be denied the ancillary drug. In other circumstances, ancillary treatment may be given to all trial participants, or only to some in standardized fashion and carefully recorded. Finally, an ancillary drug may be given "on request" as symptomatic therapy and the amount consumed may be used as a criterion for evaluating the efficacy of the test drug.

It is often necessary to plan a washout period for previously administered treatment to ensure the absence of a "carry-over" effect.

At the end of a double-blind period, if the drug administered has been effective, the problem of continuation arises. No solution is universally applicable.

The drugs compared should be labelled and packaged clearly and unambiguously so as to eliminate any possible cause of error.

The choice of a comparator is not enough to define the "Therapeutics" chapter of a study protocol. The dose and administration schedule must also be chosen.

For the comparison of two supposedly active compounds, the confrontation must be fair: for example, a new treatment should not be favored by comparing it with a proven treatment, but given at doses that are too small, less than those at which its efficacy is recognized and at which it is usually prescribed.

1. CHOICE OF DOSAGES

Before starting a controlled trial of a new compound, phase 1 studies must have determined the range of acceptable doses.

1.1. Fixed dosages

Fixed dosages are sometimes recommended with a view to standardizing the conditions of the trial and hence to reducing the variability of the response to treatment. In fact, it is more logical to consider that uniformization of treatment by using fixed dosage may actually *increase* variability since some patients will be receiving too much drug, and others not enough (5).

If a treatment under investigation is *intended to be administered at fixed dosage* (e.g. oral contraceptives or vaccines), comparative trials for such treatments are greatly simplified (once the "right" dose has been determined) and corresponds to the future therapeutic reality.

Other drugs may be prescribed without too many problems at intermediate "universal" doses which will actually be recommended later to prescribing physicians. In this case, the trial with fixed dosage answers the question "what is the efficacy compared to the standard dose of treatments?" and not to the question "what is the optimal compared efficacy of the treatments?" (6).

1.2. Dose-response relationship

Some controlled clinical trials may aim to compare *several fixed dosages* of the same drug. This type of trial determines the optimal fixed dosage but not the optimal effect achieved in each patient with his individual optimal dose. In addition, one of the requirements of such a trial is that none of the dosages tested should cause any problem of toxicity in any patient so that it can be assigned randomly. This type of trial enables study of the *dose-response relationship* (1, 4). It is also desirable to include a placebo group so that the lowest dose producing a significant difference from the placebo can be established (9, 12, 13). The range of doses investigated depends on how they are spaced out and the number of doses as discussed in chapter 1.

It is also possible to compare two treatments, using several doses of each. For example, a regimen using two doses of a treatment and three doses of another treatment has been used in a trial comparing morphine with heroin in the treatment of postoperative pain (8).

1.3. Increasing doses

1.3.1. Forced titration

In some trials, the drugs compared are administered using the same stepwise dosage increments in all subjects. This administration modality assumes that there is no carry-over effect or that an intermediate withdrawal period suffices to eliminate this effect completely, and (as below) the highest dose can be safely administered to all patients.

1.3.2. Non-forced titration

In this form of administration, dosage is increased by predetermined progressive increments, until optimal efficacy is reached, or until the development of adverse effects which are too uncomfortable. The rules governing modification of doses during a trial must always be fixed in advance. Analysis of results must take into account the cumulative probability of success according to the increase in the dose (2, 3). Adjustment of dosage can be optimized by taking into account monitoring data a priori and cumulative experience to reach pre-determined plasma levels (10).

1.4. Adjusted doses

In some comparisons of two pharmacologically active drugs, each one must be administered at its *optimum dose* (adjusted, if necessary individually in each patient), so that the comparison is *equitable. Dosage can be adjusted initially* according to weight, body surface, severity of the disorder, and plasma levels of the drug after administration of a test dose (7).

Some drugs must *necessarily be administered in adjustable doses* with close monitoring of their efficacy (e.g. anticoagulants) or their plasma levels (e.g. lithium). In such cases, a fixed dosage trial would be absurd. Subjects receiving different but still optimal dosages should not be separated in the analysis.

Since dosage adjustment is problematical under double-blind conditions, trials that include a placebo are sometimes preceded by a *trial and error approach to find the "right" dose for each patient before the double-blind phase*, and then randomly assigning the patient to receive either the active drug or the placebo.

Nevertheless, if one wants to adjust dosage under "blind conditions", it is difficult in a placebo-controlled trial to avoid escalation dose increases in the placebo group alone. This difficulty can be limited if the number of "dose increments" is no more than two or three, or if a maximum dose not to be exceeded can be set, above which superior efficacy cannot be obtained and for which there are no serious problems of toxicity. The use of an independent non-blind observer may help in resolving this difficulty. For example, when dosage adjustment is made based on a laboratory criterion that the non blind observer only knows, for each change of dose of one patient receiving the active drug, a similar change must be done for a placebo patient.

2. TIMING

The timing of drug administration (and of food intake) is often an important factor determining drug efficacy. The dosage schedule should be established as a function of the time-course of drug concentrations in biological fluids, the duration of drug effects and the time at which the criteria of response are measured.

If a supposedly active drug is compared to a placebo, the dosage schedule does not raise any problems since the placebo can always be given at the same time as the active drug.

If, on the other hand, two supposedly active drugs are being compared, their ideal schedules may be different. This problem may be overcome by using the "double-dummy" technique, and thus add up administrations, but then the treatment may become overly complicated. *If more than two drugs* have to be administered at different times, then this technique is virtually not feasible and a compromise (that carries a risk of placing one of the treatments at a disadvantage) is difficult to find.

3. CONCOMITANT TREATMENTS

Some concomitant treatments cannot be avoided, while others are part of the study objective.

3.1. Unavoidable treatments

In a clinical trial, the ideal situation would be to withdraw all other medication so that only the "pure" effects of the treatment compared could be studied. This is seldom possible with sick patients.

Two cases must be distinguished:

3.1.1. Unauthorized treatments

These are not allowed in *any* patient in the trial. If they are indispensable (or if a patient refuses to do without them), they constitute an *exclusion criterion* for patient selection.

3.1.2. Authorized treatments

Often it will be necessary to accept certain concomitant medications, in *exceptional cases*, on the condition that all treatments received by each subject in the trial be carefully recorded, and allowance must be made for such treatments when interpreting the results. In such cases, it is often possible to *standardize* symptomatic co-therapy such as hypnotics or analgesics by restricting the choice for each indication to a standard dose (fixed or adjusted e.g. on a body weight basis) of a single predetermined drug.

3.2. Concomitant treatments that are part of the trial objective

3.2.1. Systematic long term

These treatments must be administered to *all* patients, for example, psychotherapy or social counselling in trials with psychotropic drugs, and physiotherapy in trials in patients with rheumatic disease. In order not to deprive some patients of the recognized beneficial effects of concomitant medication, these treatments are prescribed for all patients and the added effect of the medication under study will be evaluated. Although this *add-on trial* has the advantage of being ethically more acceptable, it renders the demonstration of a therapeutic effect more difficult since an "additional" effect is less striking that an effect produced by single drug therapy.

3.2.2. Symptomatic treatments as requested

In some trials, the *consumption* or *frequency of use* of a symptomatic treatment in a *fail-safe trial* have been proposed as the *criterion of efficacy* for the drug under investigation: this is the case for pure analgesics in trials of anti-inflammatory drugs or nitroglycerin in trials of anti-anginal agents.

3.2.3. Fixed combination (factorial design)

Sometimes, it is possible to *simultaneously test* the effect of two treatments (that are or are not concomitant medications depending on the patient), by randomization on two levels as shown in the following example:

- first randomization: treatment A or B
- second randomization: (A + C or A + D) or (B + C or B + D) where A and B could represent the drug treatments, and C and D two types of psychotherapy

This "factorial design" makes it possible to test the interaction of concomitant treatments.

4. DISCONTINUATION OF PRIOR THERAPY

In long-term trials involving patients with chronic disease, it is seldom possible to limit recruitment to previously untreated patients. This raises the problem of discontinuing prior therapy, which can only be done if its results were deemed insufficient, otherwise there may be ethical objections to including patients in the trial.

In addition, it generally is necessary to arrange for a "washout period", the length of which will be proportional to the duration of the carry-over effect of the previous treatment.

However, if a previous treatment has caused lasting effects (e.g. amenorrhea after oral contraceptive therapy), exclusion of the patient from the trial may have to be considered, depending on the type and aim of the study.

5. CONTINUATION OR DISCONTINUATION OF TREATMENT AT THE END OF THE TRIAL

When a patient has completed the prescribed course of a randomly assigned treatment as stipulated by the trial protocol, the problem of continuing or discontinuing the treatment arises.

This problem is particularly relevant to patients with chronic disease whose condition may require continuation of treatment when the result achieved has been *satisfactory*.

There is no ideal standard solution to this problem but several possibilities can sometimes be considered.

• Systematic discontinuation of the treatments compared in all patients is the most satisfactory solution, provided replacement by an equivalent drug is both safe and possible.

• If two active drugs are being compared, and if sudden substitution of these drugs can be undertaken safely, then at the end of the trial period treatment for all patients in the trial may be be continued with one of the drugs compared by stipulating this in the protocol.

• In some trials, provision may be made for breaking the code for each individual patient at the end of his trial period. This procedure implies that all the data for evaluation of the results has been collected and validated definitively before the code has been broken, and that subsequent reevaluation of the results will not be performed nor that the validity of the data will be questioned. Otherwise, the entire double-blind design will be worthless.
One drawback of this practice is that it risks dampening the enthusiasm of the medical staff, the sponsor and the patients either already entered, (or to be recruited) from pursuing the trial, should one of the treatments compared appear to be inferior after partial evaluation. Logically, premature evaluation of intermediate results should not permit any sort of conclusion, but it is psychologically difficult to disregard a preliminary evaluation once it has been performed. This procedure, therefore, is not recommended.

• It is possible to continue the treatment prescribed in a double-blind manner during the trial period until the final code-breaking, i.e. not only at the end of the period of observation of the *last* patients entered in the trial, but also until completion of work for validation of data.

This solution poses insoluble practical problems. It must be planned in the protocol and the maximum duration of treatment must be compatible with available toxicology data on the test drug and with regulatory requirements. In addition, one does not know, when the first patient enters a trial, how much time will be necessary to recruit the planned number of subjects, the maximum duration of prolonged treatment, and thus the total amount of drug supplies to be prepared under coded packaging.

• Whether this is at the end of the trial or at the end of the double-blind period for each patient, long-term continuation of a treatment that proved to be effective in a specific subject may be problematical if the drug administered turns out to be the placebo or if it is a new drug that has produced poor overall results by virtue of which the manufacture decides to discontinue production....

6. PACKAGING AND LABELLING

Consideration should be given to appropriate packaging and labelling which should meet the following requirements (11):

- be practical and avoid dosage errors,
- facilitate compliance with treatment,
- the drug should not have an overly "experimental" appearance even for non-marketed drugs, as this may cause the patient undue concern.

When the dosage schedule of the drugs compared is different particularly if they look alike (placebo interspersed with an active drug to equalize the number of daily doses), a satisfactory solution consists of packaging each dose individually either in blister packs or in partitioned boxes.

In complex cases, these requirements can be fulfilled with difficulty by an automated system and correct packaging and labelling of the drugs should therefore be placed under the responsibility of a person who is familiar with and understands the trial protocol.

The drugs tested should be clearly labelled and should permit identification of the trial, the test drug (through a code number in a double-blind trial), the investigator, the patient categories (for a stratified trial), the period, the expiry date and the conditions for storage. The texts should be printed in the local language, and conform to local regulations.

Those persons responsible for packaging and labelling must comply with strict operating procedures to ensure that possible sources of error are avoided.

References

1 Budde M, Bauer P. Multiple test procedures in clinical dose finding studies. JAMA 1989; *84*: 792-6.

2 Chuang C. The analysis of a titration study. Statistics in Medicine 1987; *6*: 583-90.

3 Chuang-Stein C, Shih WJ. A note on the analysis of titration studies. Statistics in Medicine 1991; *10*: 323-8.

4 Dawkins HC. Multiple comparisons misused: why so frequently in response-curve studies? Biometrics 1983; *39*: 789-90.

5 Feinstein AR. Clinical Biostatistics, III, the architecture of clinical research. Clin Pharmacol Ther 1970; *11*: 432-41.

6 Hamilton M. Clinical trials in anaesthesia. Br J Anaesth 1967; *39*: 287-93.

7 Hamilton M. The methodology of trials of anti-depressants for depressed inpatients. J Internat Med Res 1975; *3*: 64-7.

8 Kaiko RF, Wallenstein SL, Rogers AG, Grabinski PY, Houde RW. Analgesic effects of heroin and morphine in cancer patients with postoperative pain. New Engl J Med 1981; *304*: 1501-5.

9 Ruber SJ. Contrasts for identifying the minimum effective dose. JAMA 1989; *84*: 816-22.

10 Sanathanan LP, Peck C, Temple R, Lieberman R, Pledger G. Randomization, PK-controlled design, and titration: an integrated approach for designing clinical trials. Drug Information Journal 1991; *25*: 425-31.

11 Spriet A, Dupin-Spriet T. a) Bonne pratique des essais cliniques des médicaments. Bâle: Karger, 1990. b) Good practice of clinical drug trials. Basel: Karger, 1992.

12 Williams DA. A test for differences between treatment means when several dose levels are compared with a zero control. Biometrics 1971; *27*: 103-17

13 Williams DA. The comparison of several dose levels with a zero control. Biometrics 1972; *28*: 519-31.

9 - Experimental designs

SUMMARY

An (experiment) clinical trial may be designed in several different ways:

• Parallel groups represent the simplest method.

• Within-patient trials allow a smaller number of subjects to be used but they require the absence of residual effects, stability of the disorder treated, and if possible, return to the initial state between treatment phases. The major designs for within-patient trials are crossover designs, latin squares and incomplete blocks.

• The matched-pair design requires the formation of pairs of comparable subjects.

• Factorial designs make it possible to take into account the effects of the treatments compared and other factors (prognostic factors, concomitant treatments) as well as various interactions.

• With the sequential design, the data can be repeatedly examined for significance, but this design often requires: pairing of subjects, a short observation period as compared to the interval between entries into the trial, and intermediate decoding of results which can influence the subsequent progress of the trial.

When choosing an experimental design, the advantages and drawbacks of each in a given situation must be taken into account (26). The necessity of reducing the variability of the results, - thus making the statistical comparison more sensitive -, and decreasing the risk of bias necessitates taking into account other factors than those directly related to the treatments compared, thus justifying choosing a more complex experimental design should this be deemed feasible in practice.

1. PARALLEL GROUPS

Clinical trials using *parallel groups* or *"completely randomized"* trials simply consists of dividing the trial subjects at random into as many groups as there are treatments.

Usually the number of patients in each group should at least be approximately equal, since for a given number of patients, the statistical comparison is most "efficient" when the groups are balanced.

The *advantage* of parallel groups is based on its simplicity, not only for organization but also for analysis. Once the selection criteria have been fulfilled, the subjects are assumed to form a homogeneous group and one relies on randomization to balance individual differences evenly, thus assuring group comparability.

The parallel group design has been accused to have the two following *drawbacks*:
- the variability of the results between randomly chosen subjects is greatest (and the efficiency of statistical comparisons is inversely proportional to the *total* variability of the groups);
- there is also a risk of error due to the formation of non-comparable treatment groups resulting from the possibility of uneven distribution of prognostic factors between groups. Random distribution of prognostic factors does not eliminate the need for verifying group comparability.

2. WITHIN-PATIENT COMPARISONS

Within-patient trials are those in which *each subject successively receives two or more treatments, in random order*. Exceptionally, with local treatments the subjects may receive treatment on *one* side only, the other side serving as a control (16, 22, 29).

2.1. Advantages and drawbacks

2.1.1. Advantages

The within-patient design offers the following advantages:

• For a comparison of similar efficacy, fewer subjects are required than in parallel group design, since each subject is "used" *several times*.

• It considers the "internal variability" of each subject compared to himself between different phases of the trial, rather than the variability between different subjects during the same phase. Indeed, in many stable chronic disorders, or in normal subjects who remain so, within-patient variability is smaller than the variability between different individuals.

2.1.2. Drawbacks

A number of drawbacks may offset these advantages:

• The within-patient design assumes that the subject's condition is stable and that from the standpoint of efficacy of the treatments administered, *comparability is better in the same patient between different treatment periods than it is between different patients during the same treatment period*. This design is obviously of little use when the planned trial period is relatively prolonged in comparison to the expected natural history of the disorder treated. Generally speaking, within-patient trials are applicable essentially to *stable conditions* for *short courses of treatment*.

• Another drawback of the within-patient design is that it assumes that none of the treatments administered during the trial period will influence the results of the following phase of treatment. Such a *delayed* or *carry-over* effect should be considered in several circumstances:

- when the treatment has an irreversible effect (such as clinical cure!),

- when there is a delayed effect that may become apparent after termination of treatment, even if the drug has been totally excreted. This is the case for the treatment of depressive illness by MAO inhibitors. A drug may have latent effects that are potentiated or revealed by the subsequent treatment,

- when excretion of the drug or one of its metabolites is slow from biological media or receptors.

In such cases, ideally, provision should be made for an *intermediate* washout period between the phases of drug administration, such as to permit total elimination of the drug, wearing-off of its effects and, if possible, return to baseline status.

In fact during a washout period that follows improvement induced by one of the drugs administered, patients frequently do not return to their initial level of symptoms, but rather to an intermediate state. This means that at the start of each treatment period, the subjects may not be as comparable to themselves as was hoped.

Not including a washout period does not solve this problem, but deliberately disregards it. However, this may be acceptable for ethical reasons when a "relapse" i.e. a return to initial status is potentially unpleasant or dangerous for the patient. When a washout period is not included in a within-patient trial, comparison should be made between symptomatic status at the end of each treatment period. No account should be taken of the events at the beginning of each period when the effects of the former treatment have not yet worn off.

- *Conditioning* of the subject (to efficacy*, inefficacy, or to adverse effects of successive treatments) and *learning experience* (patients score better in repeated tests used as criteria for efficacy). This effect is sometimes cancelled out by randomization of the order of administration.

- Conversely, a "rebound" effect may be observed by inversion of the effect when treatment is stopped, thus affecting the following phase.

Unfortunately, to detect the influence of *carry-over effects* on the results, we must use a method based on the variability *between individuals*, hence less sensitive, less "powerful" and requiring more subjects than the within-patient comparison of the treatments themselves, especially if there is a weak correlation between the responses of the two periods (34, 35). Therefore the advantage of having to enlist fewer patients is lost if we wish to make sure that there is no carry-over effect (3, 17). If there is reason to suspect a carry-over effect, the only way to salvage some of the data is to analyze the results in parallel groups for the initial period of the trial only, disregarding the subsequent "contaminated" periods (3, 9).

* This can explain differences between treatments in opposite directions before and after crossing-over.

Figure 1
Cross-over trial:
Diagrammatic representation of
"treatment" effects (T), "period"
effects (Per) and "treatment x
period" interaction (T x Per).

Figures 1a, 1b, 1c and 1d:
examples without "treatment x
period" interaction.
Figures 1e, 1f, 1g and 1h:
examples with interaction

S = severity index
t = time
I = first period
II = second period
A, B = the two treatments
compared

N.B.: figures 1e and 1f are
extreme examples: treatment
A is better than treatment B
during the first period and
treatment B is better than
treatment A during the second
period (crossover or
"qualitative" interaction).

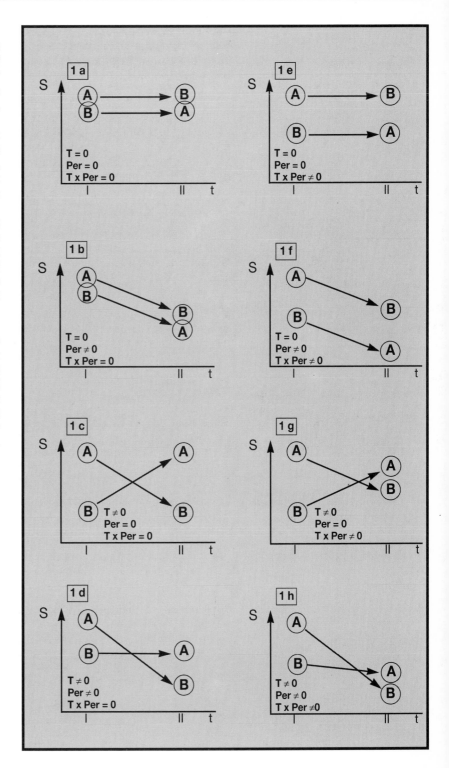

Interpretation of the results may be rendered even more difficult if, in addition to the carry-over effect, there is a "period" effect (17). For example during the second period the results are often better (or worse) than during the first period, regardless of the treatment administered.

Figure 1 is a diagrammatic representation of the possible combinations of the *"period" effect* and the *period x treatment interactions*.

Figure 2 illustrates a case of interaction obviously due to the period effect (the difference is proportional to the baseline level which changes in time). This effect can sometimes be corrected by adequate transformation of the variables.

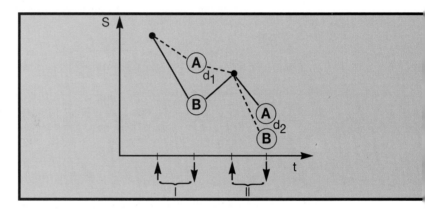

Figure 2
Cross-over trial
Period x treatment interaction due to a "period effect".
A, B: evaluation of effects of treatments A and B
d1 d2: differences between the treatments at periods I and II
S = severity index
t = time
↑ = start of a treatment
↓ = end of a treatment
I = first period
II= second period

Figure 3 shows an example of interaction clearly related to a carry-over effect. In this case, the second period cannot be used and only a "parallel group" analysis for the initial period can be performed.

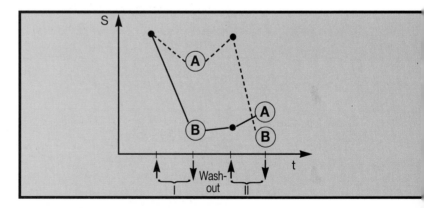

Figure 3
Cross-over trial?
Period x treatment interaction illustrating a carry-over effect (same abbreviations as in figure 2)

Many experimental designs are proposed to take carry-over effects into account:
- formation of four groups AB, BA, AA and BB
- trials with 3 or 4 periods with for example repetition of the 2nd or more complicated designs ABBA, BAAB....(6, 7, 11, 12, 14, 23, 24, 25).

In practice, within-individual trials contain a risk and it is wise to reserve them for protocols that have been shown by experience to be unassociated with a period-treatment interaction for the length of treatment and withdrawal periods of the trial considered. *This is often the case in healthy volunteers*, but rarely so in patients, even with chronic and stable conditions (30). Moreover, the interaction is often manifested by a difference between treatments, smaller during the second period than during the first. This results in an under-estimate of the difference (5).

• The total duration of observation, for each patient, is extended, with repetition of tests intended to assess efficacy and tolerability, which can result in decreased motivation and early discontinuations (some patients will not have participated in all the study periods).

2.2. The major within-patient experimental designs

2.2.1. The crossover trial

In the crossover design, two treatments A and B are compared by administering each drug to all patients in randomized order: A followed by B, or B followed by A. It is necessary to study both the effects of the treatments and *the order in which they are administered* by an appropriate statistical method.

2.2.2. Latin square design

If more than two treatments are being compared in a trial, they may be administered successively to all the participants in such a way that:

• the number of subjects is equal to the number of treatments (or to a multiple of this number);

• *each subject* successively receives *each treatment*;

• *each treatment* is administered to one of the subjects during *each successive period* of the trial.

With three treatments A, B, and C, for example, the resulting design is shown in figure 4.

Figure 4

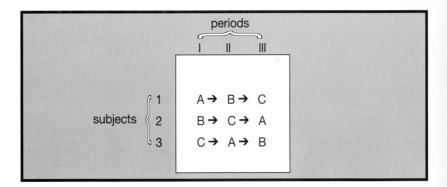

This design is called a "latin square" design because the treatments are designated by the latin letters A, B, and C.

Using this design, the influence of three factors (namely the subject, the phase and the treatment*) on the criterion of evaluation can be studied simultaneously.

If the number of subjects exceeds the number of treatments, it must be a multiple of this number: In this case several latin squares are used.

If the order in which the treatments are administered is likely to influence their efficacy, it is preferable not to use a latin square design consisting of "circular permutations" of the same letters, since this limits the succession to AB; BC, AC (and not BA, CB, AC) as in the example shown in figure 5 (easy to recognize since the same letters are found on a diagonal line).

Figure 5

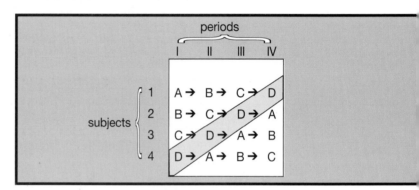

In the example illustrated in figure 6, the rows of the square (corresponding to the subjects) have been permuted. This produces the same drawbacks as in the previous example, despite the absence of diagonal alignment: figure 6

Figure 6

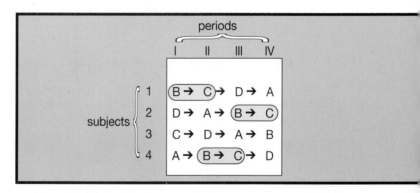

* Nevertheless, with the latin square design, it is not possible to test any "period-treatment interaction".

To avoid this drawback, we can use *latin squares balanced for the order effect* (36).

• If we are dealing with an even number of treatments, a single special latin square can be used which presents every possible order and allows estimation of the residual effects of treatments (figure 7).

Figure 7

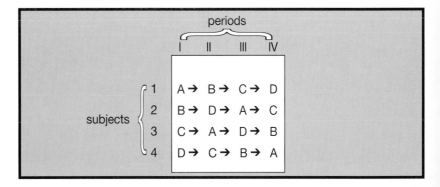

• If there are an odd number of treatments, two latin squares must be used in the particular cases of two 3 x 3 squares, they may simply be mirror-images of each other (21): figure 8.

Figure 8

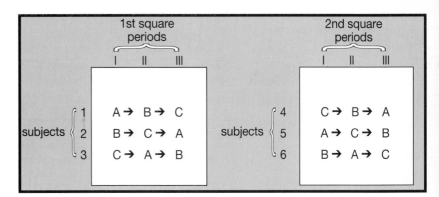

A variant of the latin square permits assessment of the difference of effect of the same treatment administered during two successive phases, by repeating the last treatment once (1) (replication of the last column): figure 9.

Figure 9

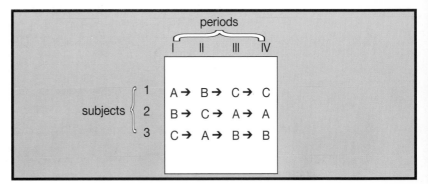

Randomization in a therapeutic trial using the latin square design is performed by successive allocation in the following manner (8):

• select a "standard" latin square (the first row and first column are made up of letters in alphabetical order) if there are several possibilities for the model chosen with the help of a latin square tables (8);

• assign each row (sequence of treatments) to a subject;

• for 6 x 6 squares or more, the periods (columns) must also be randomly permutated;

• finally, each letter used is attributed to a treatment at random.

In latin squares balanced for the order effect, the columns cannot be permutated as this may destroy the balance.

2.2.3. Greco-latin squares

If it is desired to study simultaneously the effect of treatment in each subject and the effect of other factors of which there are as many varieties as there are treatments, and which can be randomly assigned (concomitant treatment, diet, etc.) two independent or "orthogonal" latin squares (found in special tables) can be superimposed to form a "Greco-Latin Square" as shown in figure 10.

Figure 10

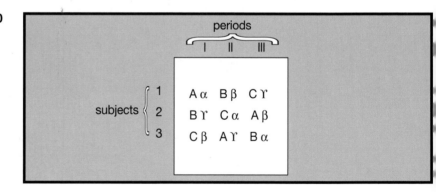

2.2.4. Incomplete blocks

To compare more than two treatments in the same subjects, each of whom cannot be given all the treatments, the latter can be arranged in incomplete blocks. For example, four treatments, A, B, C and D can be compared (33), in subjects each of whom will receive only two of the treatments (figure 11).

Figure 11

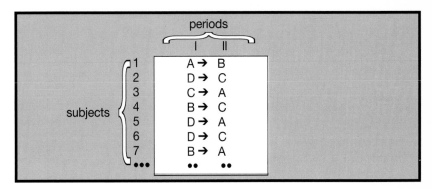

2.2.5. "Intensive" designs

An extreme type of within-patient trial has been proposed and referred to as an "intensive design" (4, 13, 20, 32). In this model, a subject receives each of the treatments compared *several times* in random order. In theory, a trial could thus be even conducted with a single subject and two or three treatments, as in the example illustrated by figure 12.

Figure 12

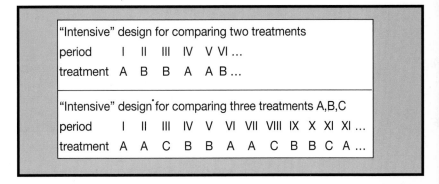

This method is applicable only for very short treatments (or even limited to a single administration) and requires a particularly cooperative subject, since the number of necessary periods to obtain a sufficient statistical power may be considerable. It may be useful for testing the efficacy of new compounds but obviously makes no claims for the representativity of the subject.

3. MATCHED PAIRS

Another method for assigning patients when comparing two treatments A and B, is to form pairs of subjects possessing, ideally, the same characteristics and who might be expected to respond similarly to the treatments.

Treatment A is then assigned randomly to one of the members of the pair and the other gets treatment B. (If more than two treatments are being compared, it is possible to form "triplets" and so on).

This method has the advantage of reducing the *difference* between subjects receiving the different treatments compared, thus decreasing intra-pair variability and imbalance. Its major drawback, however, is the *difficulty in forming well-matched pairs,* which increases as the number of characteristics for which the subjects have to be matched rises.

In practice, pairing is feasible in only three situations:

• When the number of characteristics matched is small (one or two), which means taking the risk of overlooking important factors of variability;

• When all the participants in a therapeutic trial are known *before* the trial is begun. This is often the case for trials on healthy volunteers and permits the best possible match to be made;

• In therapeutic trials on homozygous twins, but such trials are only very rarely possible (27).

4. FACTORIAL DESIGNS

When it is wished to study *simultaneously* the influence of the treatments compared and that of one or several other factors assigned by randomization as well as their interaction (2), a "factorial design" may be used.

The factor considered may involve an adjuvant treatment, a special diet (31), or the co-prescription of psychotherapy (15). This method is used especially to study drug combinations either with fixed dosage (A + B, A + Placebo of B, B + Placebo of A, Placebo of A + Placebo of B) (10, 28) or in dose-seeking trials, which in this case enables determination of the dose-response surface (three dimensional equivalent of the dose-response curve) (18, 19) (figure 13).

Figure 13

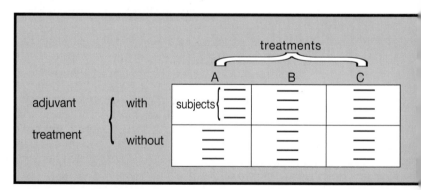

By making the statistical comparisons more sensitive and by allowing the influence of several factors to be tested at the same time (which might otherwise have required several distinct trials), the use of a factorial design *reduces the number of subjects* needed to reach a satisfactory conclusion (37).

The *disadvantage* of factorial designs arises primarily from the complexity of the experimental design itself which entails several subgroups, separate random assignment and multiple drug batches. This complexity, however, really concerns the planning stages rather than the actual conduct of the trial.

5. SEQUENTIAL DESIGNS

In a sequential trial, the results are analyzed as the trial proceeds, whenever a case or a case per treatment is completed.

The principles underlying sequential *analysis* of results will be discussed in a later chapter. A rule for discontinuing the trial should be defined with rejection either of the null hypothesis or of an alternative hypothesis. The *advantage* of this method is that a conclusion can generally be reached with less subjects than that required in a fixed-number trial.

A *disadvantage* of the procedure is that it requires reaching a definitive conclusion about one case (or a pair of cases) before admitting further subjects into the trial. The total duration of observation for individual cases must therefore be short compared to the interval between admissions. In practice, this design is applicable only to treatments of very short duration.

Another drawback of the sequential design is that the methods of analysis often address the *difference between pairs* of subjects receiving two different treatments. *Pairing* (matching for several characteristics that may influence the chance of treatment outcome), is therefore highly desirable.The formation of pairs may be delayed by the need for waiting for each subject to find an appropriate match. Aside from within-patient trials and trials in homozygous twins, pairing may turn out to be extremely difficult, if not impossible!

Moreover, sequential trials entail complete examination of the data once each case has been completed, generally with breaking of the code in "blind" trials. This carries a risk of demotivating the clinician in charge of enlisting patients who may consciously or subconsciously modify the way he selects patients after seeing intermediate results which are not sufficient to draw valid conclusions. Finally, when the "limit" of significance is approached, the clinician may find himself faced with the dilemma of either discontinuing the trial too soon or continuing to prescribe a treatment which he is persuaded places patients receiving it at a disadvantage.

References

1   Arsenault A, Lebel E, Lussier A. Gastrointestinal microbleeding in normal subjects receiving acetylsalicyclic acid, placebo, and R-803, a new antiinflammatory agent in a design balanced for residual effects. J Clin Pharmacol 1976; *16*: 473-80.

2   Brittain E, Wittes J. Factorial designs in clinical trials: the effects of non-compliance and subadditivity. Statistics in Medicine 1989; *8*: 161-71.

3   Brown BW Jr. The cross-over experiment for clinical trials. Biometrics 1980; *36*: 69-79.

4   Chassan JB. Intensive design in medical research. Pharmac Therap B 1975; *1*: 139-48.

5   Cleophas TJM. Underestimation of treatment effect in crossover trials. Angiology 1990; *41*: 673-80.

6   Ebbutt AF. Three-period crossover designs for two treaments. Biometrics 1984; *40*: 219-24.

7   Elswick RK, Uthoff VA. Non-parametric approach to the analysis of the two-treatment, two-period, four-sequence crossover model. Biometrics 1989; *45*: 663-7.

8   Fisher RA, Yates F. Statistical tables for biological, agricultural, and medical research. 6th edition. Edinburgh: Oliver and Boyd, 1963.

9   Fleiss JL. A critique of recent research on the two-treatment crossover design. Controlled Clinical Trials 1989; *10*: 237-43.

10 Gibson JM, Overall JE. The superiority of a drug combination over each of its components. Statistics in Medicine 1989; *8*: 1479-84.

11 Glass RM, Uhlenhuth EH, Matuzas W et al. Subject-own-control design in evaluating clinical antidepressant effects. J Affective Disorders 1982; *4*: 373-8.

12 Gold H, Kwit NT, Messeloff CR et al. Comparison of chlorothiazide and metalluride. New rapid method for quantitative evaluation of diuretics in bed-patients. J Am Med Assoc 1960; *173*: 745-52.

13 Guyatt GH, Heyting A, Jaeschke R et al. N of 1 randomized trials for investigating new drugs. Controlled Clinical Trials 1990; *11*: 88-100.

14 Hafner KB, Koch GG, Canada AT. Statistics in Medicine 1988; *7*: 471-81

15 Hamilton M, Hordern A, Waldrop FN, Lofft J. A controlled trial on the value of prochlorperazine, trifluoperazine, and intensive care group treatment. Br J Psychiatr 1963; *109*: 510-22.

16 Happle R, Echternacht K. Induction of hair growth in alopecia areata with DNCN. Lancet 1977; *2*: 1002-3.

17 Hills M, Armitage P. The two-period cross-over trial. Br J Clin Pharmacol 1979; *8*: 7-20.

18 Hung HMJ, Ng TH, Chi GYH, Lipicky RJ. Testing for the existence of a dose combination feating its components. Proceedings of the Biopharmaceutical Sections of the American Statistical Association, 1989

19 Hung HMJ, Ng TH, Chi GYH, Lipicky RJ. Response surface and factorial designs for combination anti-hypertensive drugs. Drug Information Journal 1990; *24*: 371-8.

20 Jaeschke R, Guyatt GH. Randomized trials in the study of anti-hypertensive drugs. American Journal of Hypertension 1990; *3*: 811-4.

21 Jones B, Kenward MG. Designs and analysis of cross-over trials. London: Chapman and Hall, 1989.

22 Kragballe K, Gjertsen BT, de Hoop D et al. Double-blind right/left comparison of calcipotriol and betamethasone valerate in treatment of psoriasis vulgaris. Lancet 1991; *337*: 193-6.

23 Laska E, Meisner M. A variational approach to optimal two-treatment crossover desings: application ot carryover-effect models. J Amer Statist Assoc 1985; *80*: 704-10.

24 Laska E, Meisner M, Kushner HB. Optimal crossover designs in the presence of carryover effects. Biometrics 1983; *39*: 1087-91.

25 Matthews JNS. Optimal crossover designs for the comparison of two treatments in the presence of carryover and auto-correlated errors. Biometrika 1987; *74*: 311-20.

26 Maxwell C. The choice of design for clinical trials. Clinical Trials Journal 1968; *5*: 1139-43.

27 Miller JZ, Nance WE, Norton JA, Wolen RL, Griffith RS, Rose RJ. Therapeutic effect of vitamin C. A co-twin control study. J Amer Med Assoc 1977; *237*: 248-9.

28 Motolese M, Muisan C, Colombi A. Hypotensive effect of oxprenolol in mild to moderate hypertension: a multicentre controlled study. Europ J Clin Pharmacol 1975; *8*: 21-31.

29 Rosner B. Statistical methods in ophthalmology. An adjustment for the intraclass correlation between eyes. Biometrics 1982; *38*: 105-14.

30 Sever PS, Poulter NR, Bulpitt CS. Double-blind crossover versus parallel groups in hypertension. Am Heart J 1989; *117*: 735-9.

31 Truelove SC. Stilboestrol, phenobarbitone, and diet in chronic duodenal ulcer. A factorial therapeutic trial. Br Med J 1960; 559-66.

32 Uhlenhuth EH, Turner DA, Purchatzke G, Gift T, Chassan J. Intensive design in evaluating anxiolytic agents. Psychopharmacology 1977; *52*: 79-85.

33 Westlake WJ. The use of balanced incomplete block designs in comparative bioavailability trials. Biometrics 1974; *30*: 319-27.

34 Willan AR. Using the maximum test statistic in the two-period cross-over clinical trial. Biometrics 1988; *44*: 211-8.

35 Willan AR, Pater JL. Carryover and the two-period cross-over clinical trial. Biometrics 1986; *42*: 593-9.

36 Williams EJ. Experimental designs balanced for the estimation of residual effects of treatments. Austral J Sc Res 1949; *1*: 149-68.

37 Wittenborn JR. The design of clinical trials. In: Levine J, Schiele BC, Bouthilet L. eds. Principles and problems in establishing the efficacy of psychotropic agents. Public Health Service Publication 1971; *No. 2138*: 227-62.

10 - Subjects lost to follow-up

SUMMARY   *A patient may discontinue his participation in a clinical trial, and he then becomes "lost to follow-up".*

Every effort should be made to determine the causes and promoting factors (often combined).

Treatment-related causes include :
• a preliminary therapeutic or tolerability result considered to be inadequate,
• recovery or sufficient improvement,
• poor acceptance of treatment.

Causes that are independent of treatment may be related to the trial (diagnostic procedures, too many visits) or to coincidental events. However, despite careful investigation, the cause often remains unknown.

Patients lost to follow-up decrease the information available, and thus reduce the sensitivity of the comparison and may also bias the results.

The following techniques may help to prevent the "loss" of patients :
• non-inclusion of uncooperative, non-motivated, unstable or negligent patients,
• motivation of the patient, his family and the medical and nursing staff,
• organization of a practical system of appointments for the patients,
• choice of an optimal trial length.

Incomplete cases may be included for evaluation using various "palliative" systems of analysis, but the choice is difficult since none of these systems is entirely satisfactory.

In the course of a clinical trial, some of the subjects included cannot, for various reasons, be evaluated at the end of the period stipulated in the protocol. These subjects "lost to follow-up"* create a problem for the correct evaluation of the treatments compared.

There are a certain number of preventive measures that can be taken to reduce the number of subjects lost to follow-up. Investigators should be familiar with them even if all cannot be applied in every situation.

Finally, including incomplete cases in the analysis of the results, although possible, raises difficult problems and it must always be planned in advance.

1. CAUSES

The maximum amount of information should be collected for incomplete cases, with the help of a pre-established questionnaire. Whenever possible, the patient himself should be questioned (which sometimes means calling on him at home), or alternately his doctor. In addition, a national patient identification number, in some countries, makes it possible to find out the date of death of deceased subjects, even long after the trial has ended.

It will thus be possible to analyze the cause or causes, or the factors that contributed to the subjects' losses and to make decisions regarding the analysis of results. In the report of study results, the number and causes of losses will have to be specified. It is important to make a distinction between causes that are related to the treatment and those unrelated to treatment (13).

1.1. Treatment-related causes

Causes of sample attrition related to the treatment are the most problematical since they may distort the comparison being made. There are a number of treatment-related events :

• Therapeutic efficacy or tolerability may be considered to be poor:
- either by the patient (who may discontinue the treatment and then fail to show up for evaluation on the planned date or who may go to another doctor);
- or by the physician who may consider it unjustified to pursue treatment and follow-up in a given patient.

• The therapeutic result may be so good that:
The patient (or his physician) consider it superfluous to continue treatment and follow-up.

• The treatment may be poorly accepted by the patient :
He may judge that it is too difficult to follow, too inconvenient or too unpleasant, or cause fear or boredom.

* Confusion due to ambiguous wording is frequent (drop-outs, withdrawals, missing). It is useful to distinguish the following :
• subjects, who stop their treatment but followed it as planned (see next chapter),
• Subjects lost to follow-up (this chapter),
• Subjects who were late entries in the trial and who, at the end of the trial, have had a short follow-up, and who will be discussed later in a "life-table" analysis,
• Subjects temporarily lost to follow-up who have subsequently returned, and whom we shall consider as missing data (14),
• Subjects excluded from enrollment (chapter 3),
• Cases taken out from analysis of results.

1.2. Causes unrelated to treatment

Causes unrelated to treatment may be:

• related to the trial: diagnostic procedures considered as too frequent unpleasant, or restrictive. Compliance with the protocol upsets the patient's life-style. Reception in the study center may be considered as cold.

• Related to random events: the patient may fall victim to an accident, and intercurrent illness, or undergo surgery. He may move away, forget to come to an appointment, or be unable to attend because of a transportation strike, etc.

In all these situations, one should always ask the following question: *"Had the efficacy of the treatment been different, would the occurrence of these events have been affected?"*

When the reason for the patient's withdrawal of the trial has been determined, it should not be hastily declared that the cause is unrelated to treatment. Indeed, the treatment may be indirectly and sometimes very subtly responsible for the patient's failure to remain in the trial. In addition, sometimes there simultaneously is *another cause* which may be related to the treatment.

1.3. Unknown causes

Patients followed in a clinical trial sometimes fail to keep their appointments for no apparent reason. In such cases, an inquiry should be undertaken but in some cases the cause will remain unknown. Such a case involves a subject who is *completely* lost to follow-up, while in the preceding cases, a certain amount of information could be obtained.

2. CONTRIBUTORY FACTORS

Whatever the causes of subjects being lost to follow-up, a number of factors contribute to their frequency:

• The length of the observation period

The longer the trial period, the greater the number of subjects lost to follow-up. For very long trials, an estimate should be made of the sample attrition expected to be taken into account in the calculation of the sample size.

• The characteristics of the patient population

it appears to be a reasonable assumption that the "reliable" and "unreliable" patients might differ in their psychological profiles or in other characteristics. In fact, studies that have addressed this question have failed to reach clear conclusions (3, 18).

• The investigator's attitude (3, 4, 18)

The doctor-patient relationship is a decisive factor in persuading the patient to return for subsequent evaluation. Compliance with instructions is better when the patient's personal concerns, particularly the symptom or symptoms for which he sought medical advice in the first place, are given due attention (18).

• Family, friends and the hospital environment are also factors that may contribute to the patient's judgment concerning the need for treatment, follow-up and evaluation and his consent.

3. CONSEQUENCES

3.1. Introduction of bias

Sample attrition may affect the *comparability* of the groups by reducing the information on subjects for whom the prognosis was initially more severe in one group than in another. It is therefore important to check comparability between groups *initially*, with all the subjects randomized (this verifies the efficacy of the randomization procedure) and *at the end* of the trial, with only those patients who have completed the trial (to ensure that the comparison is valid in case analysis on completers is considered (13, 15).

Subjects lost to follow-up may distort the proportion of favorable results in one of the groups if, for example, the patients who withdrew were those who had a poor result. More serious still would be a situation in which one group lost patients who had a poor result while another lost patients who had a good result (17).

If subjects are lost to follow-up as a result of a high proportion of adverse events, a bias should be suspected regarding the assessment of results for the only remaining patients since tolerability and therapeutic outcome are often linked.

3.2. Less "powerful" comparison

Regardless of the method for processing data :
- analysis of only the remaining patients,
- intention to treat analysis with replacement score,
- sensitivity analysis comparing the results of the two preceding methods,
- some information is always lost. Comparison is then less sensitive to the differences between treatments. There will be less chance of observing a "significant" difference and the "power" of the comparison is diminished.

In some instances, as many as half of the patients enlisted, or even more, may fail to complete the trial (8).

In extreme situations, comparison of the patients remaining becomes totally meaningless.

3.3. Difficulties in analyzing and interpreting results

Incomplete cases may create additional difficulties when it comes to analyzing data :

• In within-patient trials (i.e. one in which each patient successively receives each of the treatments compared), if a patient is lost between two treatments it may be difficult to interpret the data, even for the completed treatment periods (cross-over trials, latins squares, incomplete blocks).

• Similarly, when a matched-pair design is used, if one of the members of a pair drops out, the data on the other member may be worthless.

• For factorial designs, in which each combination of factors is represented by a single subject, if that patient disappears, it leaves a "gap" which may make statistical analysis difficult or even impossible under the conditions originally laid down.

4. PREVENTION

The need for keeping losses to follow-up to a minimum must be kept in mind when selecting patients for, and organizing the technical aspects of a trial. The preventive measures that can be taken derive from the causes of sample attrition:

• The subjects selected should be those who are able and willing to cooperate. However, if recruitment is confined to such patients, then the results of the trial can only be extrapolated to "cooperative" patients. In practice, it is customary to exclude only patients who are manifestly unstable or negligent, or those whose occupation entails frequent moving;

• Motivation of subjects in the trial should be ensured by explaining all aspects of the trial to them as clearly as possible, and by welcoming them as research partners;

• An attempt should be made to achieve motivation of all members of the medical and nursing staff, which may be difficult in overburdened hospital departments;

• Follow-up visits in the outpatient clinic should be made convenient for patients (5) through effective organization of appointments (19), minimal waiting time, memorandums and even reminder letters or telephone calls (1, 6);

• Repetitive, inconvenient or unpleasant tests should be reduced to a minimum as they tend to discourage both the patients and the medical staff;

• The optimal duration of treatment (13) should be sufficient to demonstrate efficacy to satisfy the objectives of the trial without waiting until the sample attrition becomes problematical. A previous trial or pilot study may serve as a guide in this choice;

• Sample size can be increased at the planning phase to compensate for attrition (16, 22).

5. ANALYSIS OF RESULTS

5.1. Description

The following items are necessary in all cases :

• The number of subjects lost in each treatment group should be clearly presented together with time of loss from the start of treatment (10);

• The cause (or causes) of each case of attrition must be determined and compared in the different treatment groups;

• The incidence of losses in each of the treatment groups must be compared. If the frequency is clearly higher in one of the treatment groups, a bias must be suspected and the results should be interpreted cautiously. it may even become necessary to abandon any statistical comparison;

• The frequency of causes in each treatment group must be compared;

• All cases should be included for the comparison of adverse effects, even if treatment was administered for only part of the time originally planned;

• If comparisons involving the completers are planned, the comparability before and after sample attrition must be verified;

• If characteristics of remaining patients are different from those of withdrawals, an effort should be made to determine whether the tendency to withdraw is related to a given characteristic.

5.2. Considering losses to follow-up in the analysis of results

The results of a trial should be analyzed using all the available data. If some of these data are incomplete, then there is no truly satisfactory solution; however, in some cases, a "lesser evil" solution can be found.

The "intention to treat" attitude consists in considering all randomized cases in the analysis including incomplete and imperfect cases (subjects lost to follow-up, non-compliers and protocol violations). For the subjects lost to follow-up, a score has to be assigned for the missing period. Intention to treat, which has a more general scope, is described in detail in chapter 14.

5.2.1. Exclusion of subjects lost to follow-up

The analysis involving only the remaining patients can be used solely if it can be recognized that patients lost to follow-up occurred randomly, i.e. in a manner totally independent of the treatment administered and its result, i.e. in exceptional cases.

A particular case is sometimes acceptable: the exclusion of a small number of randomized subjects lost to follow-up but who did not receive any dose of treatment assigned or who had no evaluation while being treated.

On the other hand, if the disappearance of a patient is due to an "end-point" used as a criterion of response to treatment (for example, death), and it occurs *between randomization and the start of treatment*, the difficulty is obvious. If a case is excluded, there is a risk of introducing bias (by eliminating one of the sickest patients from one group); if it is incorporated in the results, the patients are compared according to the treatment prescribed, and not received, which obviously has no relation to real efficacy of this treatment. If several observations of this phenomenon occur, and if by bad luck they all involve the same treatment (21), it may be very difficult to interpret the results.

5.2.2. Replacing non-completed cases

It has been suggested that drop-outs should be replaced by enlisting other patients in the same group (with the same treatment) for the trial. It can immediately be seen that this approach carries a risk. If, for example, patients who drop out of one group are those who would have had a poor result, admitting new patients into this group means that potentially favorable cases will be over-represented in this group. We are thus introducing a selection bias and this will distort the comparison to the advantage of the group in which drop-outs have been replaced.

In practice, withdrawals can be replaced only in trials involving healthy volunteers, particularly in pharmacokinetic studies, cautiously and after investigation.

5.2.3. Optimal utilization of incomplete cases

If it is considered that a comparison restricted to completed cases is too inaccurate (most frequent case), it becomes necessary to include non-completed cases.

Several palliative procedures have been proposed to use available information with the utmost efficacy. To avoid any ambiguity, it is recommended to plan the method chosen before the start of the trial and to mention it either in the protocol or in a written procedure.

• *One possibility is to analyze the data on a simple success or failure basis* (17). In this case, if a patient discontinued the trial because of improvement such that pursual of treatment was judged superfluous, he will be included among the successes. Conversely, if a patient discontinued treatment because it was judged ineffective on preliminary assessment, he will be included among the failures. One must be aware, however, that this dichotomous "black and white" classification considerably reduces the information derived from the data collected.

• The number of withdrawals may be used as a major or secondary criterion for treatment efficacy (7, 13). Subjects lost to follow-up may also serve to compare patient acceptance of the treatments under study.

• Patients may be classified in order of increasing efficacy (9) using both information on subjects lost to follow-up and discontinuation of treatment followed: discontinuations due to lack of efficacy, *then* discontinuations because of lack of tolerability, *then* final results available in order of increasing efficacy, and *finally* withdrawals because of "recovery".

• A failure score may be used in place of missing scores: the worst score observed during the time the patient was in the trial or even the score before treatment (11, 12).

• In studies where the duration of treatment is not the same for all patients between inclusion and end-point (death, recovery, recurrence, complication) patients lost to follow-up can be taken into account for the period during which they were under observation. This type of study which includes a "life-table analysis" will be discussed later.

• The missing final score may be replaced by the best score obtained among remaining patients, if losses occurred as a result of clinical improvement or recovery.

• The missing results may be replaced by a given percentile score of the patients who completed the trial, ranked in order of efficacy (for example, the 95th *percentile* which is the limit between the 95% best and the 5% worst results) (23).

• It is possible to estimate the score of an incomplete case either based on completed cases or according to available data in the case of subjects lost to follow-up. This statistical estimation of missing data should only be performed cautiously knowing and specifying the underlying assumptions that it implies.

A solution often suggested consists in taking the last available score during treatment as either the final value or the intermediate value (2, 9). This method (Last Observation Carried Forward: LOCF) is acceptable under three conditions:
- that few subjects have been lost to follow-up,
- that the method and the values carried forward are described in the trial report,
- and especially that the intermediate scores are predictive of later score (absence of tachyphylaxis, rebound or relapse effect for the disorder and therapeutic class considered).

5.2.4. Sensitivity analysis carried forward

This method consists in comparing results of two analyses based on opposite choices, for example:
- remaining cases and intention to treat,
- method of extreme bias which consider the subjects lost to follow-up for a treatment as success and the other as failures, and conversely (20).

This approach makes it possible to verify the robustness of the analysis with the options chosen.

References

1   Bigby JA. Appointment reminders to reduce no-show rates. A stratified analysis of their cost-effectiveness. JAMA 1983; *250*: 1742-5.

2   Evans SJW. What can we do with the data we throw away? Br J Clin Pharmac 1982; *14*: 653-9.

3   Fiester AR, Rudestam KE. Multivariate analysis of the early drop-out process. Consulting Clinical Psychology 1975; *43*: 528-35

4   Finnerty FA Jr, Mattie EC, Finnerty FA. Hypertension in the inner city. I. Analysis of clinic drop-outs. Circulation 1973; *47*: 73-5.

5   Finnerty FA Jr, Mattie EC, Finnerty FA. Hypertension in the inner city. II. Detection and follow-up. Circulation 1973; *47*: 76-8.

6   Fletcher SW, Appel FA, Bourgeois MA. Management of hypertension. Effect of improving patient compliance for follow-up care. JAMA 1975; *233*: 242-4.

7   Friedman AS. Interaction of drug therapy with marital therapy in depressive patients. Arch Gen Psych 1975; *32*: 619-37.

8   Glick BS. Drop-out in an out-patient, double-blind drug study. Psychosomatics 1965; *6*: 44-8.

9   Gould AL. A new approach to the analysis of clinical drug trials with withdrawals. Biometrics 1980; *36*: 721-7.

10 Hamptom JR. Presentation and analysis of the results of clinical trials in cardiovascular disease. Br Med J 1981; *282*: 1371-3.

11 Hohn R, Gross GM, Gross M, Lasagna L. A double-blind comparison of placebo and imipramine in the treatment of depressed patients in a state hospital. J Psychiat Res 1962; *1*: 76-91.

12 Lasagna L. Analgesic methodology: a brief history and commentary. J Clin Pharmacol 1980; *20*: 373-6.

13 Lasky JL. The problem of sample attrition in controlled treatment trials. J Nerv Ment Dis 1962; *135*: 332-7.

14 O'Brian Smith E, Hardy RJ, Cutter GR. A two-compartment regression model applied to compliance in a hypertension treatment program. J Chronic Dis 1980; *33*: 645-51.

15 Overall JE, Hollister LE, Pokorny AD, Casey JF, Katz G. Drug therapy in depression. Clin Pharmacol Ther 1962; *3*: 16-22.

16 Palto M, McHugh R. Adjusting for losses to follow-up in sample size determinations for cohort disease. J Chron Dis 1979; *32*: 315-26.

17 Rickels K, Boren R, Stuart HM. Controlled psychopharmacological research in general practice. J New Drugs 1964; *4*: 138-47.

18 Rosenberg CM, Rayner AE. Drop-outs from treatment. Can Psychiatr Ass J 1973; *18*: 229-33.

19 Sackett DL, Haynes RB, Gibson ES et al. Randomized clinical trial of strategies for improving medication compliance in primary hypertension. Lancet 1975; *i*: 1205-7.

20 Schwartz D, Lellouch J. Les manquants dans l'essai thérapeutique. Biometrics 1967; *23*: 145-52.

21 Shaw IW, Cornfield J, Cole CM. Statistical problems in the design of clinical trials and interpretation of results. In: Thrombosis: pathogenesis and clinical trials. IV International congress of thrombosis and hemostasis. Stuttgart: Schattauer-Verlag 1973.

22 Shork MA, Remington RD. The determination of sample size in treatment-control comparisons for chronic disease studies in which drop-out or non-adherence is a problem. J Chron Dis 1967; *20*: 233-9.

23 Simon P, Fermanian J, Ginestet D, Goujet MA, Peron-Magnan P. Standard and long-acting depot neuroleptics in chronic schizophrenia. Arch Gen Psych 1978; *35*: 893-7.

11 - Patient compliance and discontinuation of treatment

SUMMARY

Patient compliance with therapy should not be overestimated. During a clinical trial, it is a good practice to evaluate compliance by discussing it with the patient, counting unconsumed pills, supervising administration, incorporation of a urinary marker, performing assays for the drug in biological fluids, or the use of packaging designed for recording drug administrations.

Compliance depends on many factors including the illness treated, the patient's personality (confidence, motivation, awareness of the seriousness of the disease), the complexity of the prescription, the apparent efficacy, the physician's attitude and communication ability and environmental factors.

The main strategies for improving compliance are: a simple and practical therapy, an effort to convince the patient of the necessity for treatment, the use of memory aids, and the exclusion of uncooperative patients from the study...

Compliance should be taken into account when analyzing the results: by a comparison of compliance rates for each treatment studied, by the comparison of results (efficacy and tolerability) in compliant and non-compliant patients, by discussion of results according to compliance, and by increasing the number of patients in the trial if the expected compliance rate is low.

In a therapeutic trial it is often assumed (at least implicitly) that patients will take the therapy that has been assigned to them exactly as prescribed. In fact, for many patients this is not the case. Although prescribers generally believe that this problem does not concern *their* patients, they are almost always wrong. Patient *compliance* rates are consistently overestimated and studies that have addressed the question have shown that 30 to 50% of patients do not take the prescribed drugs properly. The magnitude of the problem is such that it cannot be ignored. Consequently, when conducting a clinical trial, the extent of the problem should be evaluated, contributory factors determined and, as far as possible, means of preventing non-compliance envisaged. The phenomenon of non-compliance must also be taken into account for the analysis of the results (6).

Non-compliance with therapy may diminish the differences in treatment efficacy or toxicity, or it may distort these differences by introducing a bias if non-compliance is more prevalent in one treatment group than in another. Furthermore, for a given non-compliance rate, the less effective treatment is at an advantage. This is particularly relevant to trials comparing an active drug with a placebo, where non-compliance favors the placebo.

Occasionally, it may be discovered that some patients are taking more, and sometimes much more than the prescribed dose. It has even been found that patients were mistakenly given one of the treatments compared but not the one which was assigned to them by the randomization procedure (12, 42).

1. MEASURING COMPLIANCE

There is no simple and infallible method for measuring the true amount of drug taken by a given patient, nor for determining if the drug was really taken as prescribed. It is desirable, nevertheless, to estimate compliance using one or more of the available methods, even though none of them are fool-proof. These methods include: questioning the patient, counting the number of doses left over, and performing assays to detect the drug or a tracer in biological fluids. On the basis of this evaluation, we may classify patients as very good, good or fair "compliers" (the significance of each of these grades must be specified in the protocol) (14). Alternatively, we may determine the number of doses omitted or the number of days without treatment for each individual patient.

Regardless of the method used, it is desirable to explain it to the patient so that he can participate in the trial with confidence. This doesn't mean spying on him but rather the evaluation of "always imperfect" compliance.

1.1. Questioning the patient

Questioning the patient is the most straightforward method for determining how well the drug was taken. However, the interview must be conducted with tact and understanding, if honest answers are to be obtained (14, 17). A reprehensive attitude by the investigator can often produce false answers. The simplest approach is to ask the patient, during each follow-up visit, how many times he forgot to take the drug, and to record his answer on the individual report form.

However, confronting the patients' answers with the amount of drug left over has shown that compliance is often overestimated by the direct method (17).

1.2. Pill count

When the trial participants are outpatients, each subject is asked to return any drug left over at each follow-up visit, thus allowing the amount of unused drug to be determined. It thus is possible to count the drug left over, knowing obviously that the amount of drug missing has not necessarily be taken, nor used in accordance with the instructions. By providing patients with bottles containing surplus tablets (or capsules, etc.), there should be some remaining at the next visit. A good correlation has been demonstrated between the results obtained by pill counts and those of tracer studies (30). The simple fact of returning or forgetting to return unused drug may be considered as a measure of compliance and appears to correlate satisfactorily with the detection of a tracer.

1.3. Supervising drug intake

The nursing staff may be asked to supervise compliance with therapy in inpatients by having the patients take the drug in the nurses' presence. However, one can never be absolutely sure that a patient has really swallowed a tablet and there have been documented cases, particularly in the psychiatric setting, of patients forcing themselves to vomit to eliminate a drug they had swallowed. Finally, the occasional presence of an observer may temporarily modify a subject's behavior. All of these items account for the fact that the results of this technique correlate poorly with urinary tracer assays (2).

1.4. Detecting a "tracer"

The addition to the drug of a small amount of a tracer substance, easy to detect in the urine, provides a relatively simple method for monitoring self-administration of drugs. The tracer used must possess a number of properties: it must be pharmacologically inert, safe, and it must not react chemically with the drug under study. Several substances have been advocated for this purpose including phenol red, trace amounts of isoniazid (10), fluorescein, riboflavin, bromide (30), or phenobarbital (29). One of the major weaknesses of this procedure is that it only provides information about the *most recent dose* taken, which may be the only one taken (patient feeling guilty just before a follow-up visit) or the only one forgotten (in the rush to get to the hospital on time or because the patient was asked to come fasting). Furthermore, in some cases a special drug formulation may have to be prepared, and this entails a risk of altered bioavailability.

1.5. Assaying the drug in biological fluids

Plasma or urinary drug levels also carry the disadvantage of only reflecting the most recent intake of drug and are, in addition, generally difficult to perform technically and not applicable to placebo. They are sometimes used for spot-checks in patients and at times chosen at random. Plasma levels are sometimes determined for a totally different reason, namely to study the correlation between plasma levels and efficacy.

1.6. Automatic recording of daily intakes

Pharmaceutical dispensing devices are available which contain an electronic circuit for recording the times when dose units are taken (1, 4, 8, 9, 32, 43). After computer processing of the information recorded, these devices make it possible not only to measure overall compliance between two visits but also to assess the regularity of compliance over time, something that is important in many therapeutic schedules (5, 33). They also enable the detection of temporary overconsumption of a drug which may be the cause of intolerance.

However, there have been instances when this system was activated.... and the drug was discarded! Yet, it is difficult to imagine that this can occur systematically and often.

1.7. Simultaneous use of these procedures

These methods are not mutually exclusive. In particular, in a *placebo versus active drug trial*, it may be wise to assay either the drug under study (for the *active drug*) or a tracer added to the placebo only. In this case, it must be ensured that the person performing the assays does not break the double blind code e.g. by informing the clinician on more than the compliance itself.

2. CAUSES AND PROMOTING FACTORS OF NON-COMPLIANCE

The causes of non-compliance with treatment may be classified into causes related to the illness under study, patient characteristics, the treatment or its effects, the medical staff and external conditions.

2.1. The illness

The non-compliance rate varies from one illness to another (13, 23) and appears to be higher when the potential risk resulting from the illness is perceived to be small by the patient, although not all studies agree on this point (31).

2.2. The subject

Few convincing relationships have been found between treatment compliance and demographic determinants such as age, sex, or intelligence (13, 19). However, comprehension of the instructions may be affected by language problems. It has not been possible to clearly establish a typical profile for the compliant and non-compliant patient, but his motivation, awareness of the seriousness of the illness and confidence in the treatment appear to be important determinants for compliance with therapy.

2.3. The treatment

The *complexity* of a treatment, particularly the number of drugs prescribed (23, 39), and the number of daily doses (9), appear to be important factors in determining compliance with therapy. The *duration* of treatment (15) probably also plays an important role; patients tend to take the treatment properly at the beginning, and as time goes by an "attrition" phenomenon sets in.

How the patient judges the efficacy of treatment may also be an important determinant of compliance. He may consider himself cured and stop treatment or he may discontinue taking the treatment because he feels it is ineffective and therefore pointless. The role of side-effects appears to vary from one study to another (15, 27, 40), but does not seem to be very important provided patients are forewarned of their possible occurrence (27).

2.4. The investigator and his staff

The physician-patient relationship often has a considerable influence on compliance with treatment. Compliance rates are clearly higher when the physician is kind and understanding, shows concern for the patients' problems and is easy to communicate with (23).

2.5. The environment

The setting in which treatment is administered has a considerable influence on compliance. Inpatients generally comply better than outpatients.

3. STRATEGIES FOR IMPROVING PATIENT COMPLIANCE WITH TREATMENT

Most of the strategies that can be used for improving compliance can in fact be extended beyond the scope of clinical trials and this may justify their use even if the trial is designed to study the results of treatment under the *true conditions of drug intake*. The very strategies used for improving patient compliance with therapy have themselves been tested in controlled trial to determine their usefulness (11, 17, 20, 21, 22, 25, 35, 36).

The major strategies that can be suggested are as follows:

• Simplification of the *treatment*, consisting of a small number of daily doses (22), easy-to-recognize tablets to eliminate the risk of confusion in case of concomitant medications (39,41), practical unit packaging especially adapted for the treatment prescribed and for the times of administration (11, 37).

• Every effort should be made to *convince* the patient of the need for treatment (28) by explaining the details of the trial to him in lay terms (20). It is also useful to provide the patient with an explanatory leaflet and to inform him of possible side-effects (27).

• The patient may be given *memory aids* in the form of a calendar consisting of detachable sheets or self-adhesive labels that should be displayed in a clearly visible location in the patient's home or office (24).

• The exclusion criteria should be extended to cover uncooperative patients who are expected not to take their treatment as prescribed. Such a selection process raises the problem of lack of "representativeness" of the subjects included in the trial (14). Participants thus selected no longer represent a sample of the patient population to which we wish to generalize the results.

The problem can only be solved if the aim of the trial is clearly defined: are we comparing treatments under "ideal conditions" or under "usual conditions"?

4. TAKING COMPLIANCE INTO ACCOUNT IN THE ANALYSIS OF THE RESULTS

Evaluation of compliance for each trial participant provides useful information in the analysis of results.

4.1. Excluding "non-compliers" from the analysis of results is generally not recommended since this would mean that the remaining groups could no longer be considered as having been formed at random and a bias may thus be introduced due to the elimination of subjects with "different" characteristics (34). Therefore, an analysis by *intention to treat* (regardless of the actual treatment taken) is always important even if other analyses sorting out "non-compliers" look useful.

4.2. The compliance rates for the treatments under study *must be compared*. This comparison may be considered to reflect the *acceptance* of the treatments and may partly account for differences in efficacy and tolerability.

4.3. Another important point *to compare* is *tolerability* and *efficacy*, between compliers and non-compliers within each treatment group (26, 38). To do this we must define what we mean by compliers and non-compliers (in the study protocol) and we must be aware of the fact that 100% compliance in long trials is very seldom achieved. We may, for example, be content to define compliers as patients who have taken at least 75% of the prescribed drug.

4.4. Finally, it is necessary to take into account the anticipated compliance rate for the type of patient studied so as not to overestimate the difference in efficacy which one seeks to detect and to adjust the number of patients enlisted to the *number needed for the trial* (16,18).

4.5. However, it is wise to be cautious with reference to the methods of *adjustment of efficacy comparisons taking compliance* as a *covariate*. Indeed, compliance measured after randomization is not a really baseline feature of the subject and can itself be influenced by efficacy (16).

5. WITHDRAWALS FROM TREATMENT

Definitive termination of treatment can occur under different circumstances.

5.1. A decision made by the patient

In some cases, it is the patient (or his family doctor), who unbeknown to the investigator, decides to discontinue the treatment, although possibly rightly, if for example, tolerability is inadequate. The patient may judge that it is unnecessary to undergo later tests in the trial. He then comes under the heading of losses to follow-up as discussed in the preceding chapter. In all cases, every effort must be made to follow him up, first to ensure the patient's own safety, and second to obtain the information necessary for analysis by "intention to treat".

5.2. A decision made by the investigator

In other cases, it is the investigator who decides to discontinue treatment because of an unfavorable course. Here too, every effort must be made to complete the tests stipulated in the protocol, both for the patients' sake and for the study data which will permit the best possible analysis of these cases.

5.3. Discontinuations planned for by the protocol

It is possible to use discontinuations of treatment as a criterion of response. Each patient continues the treatment under study as long as efficacy or tolerability is justified. If not, treatment is discontinued. A replacement medication is prescribed. Statistical comparison then involves the *duration* of administration of the treatments compared by using the "life-table" method (3, 7).

References

1 Averbuch M, Weintraub M, Pollock DJ. Compliance assessment in clinical trials. The MEMS device. J Clin Res Pharmacoepidemiol 1990; *4*: 190-204.

2 Ballinger BR, Ramsay AC, Stewart ML. Methods of assessment of drug administration in a psychiatric hospital. Br J Psychiat 1975; *127*: 494-8

3 Capell HA, Rennie JAN, Rooney PJ et al. Patient compliance: a novel method of testing non-steroidal antiinflammatory analgesics in rheumatoid arthrosis. J Pharmacol 1979; *6*: 584-93.

4 Cheung R, Dickins J, Nicholson PW et al. Compliance with antituberculous therapy: a field trial of a pill-box with a concealed electronic recording device. Eur J Clin Pharmacol 1988; *35*: 401-7.

5 Cramer JA, Scheyer RD, Mattson RH. Compliance declines between clinic visits. Arch Intern Med 1990; *150*: 1509-10.

6 Cramer JA, Spilker B. Patient compliance in medical practice and clinical trials. New-York: Raven Press, 1991.

7 Delbarre F, Mery C. Evaluation de l'effet au long cours des médicaments antirhumatismaux par la méthode des taux de poursuite. C R Acad Sc Paris 1980; *290*: série D 45-8.

8 Eisen S A, Hanpeter JA, Kreuger LW, Gard M. Monitoring medication compliance: description of a new device. Compliance in Health Care 1987; *2*: 131-42.

9 Eisen SA, Millers DK, Woodward RS et al. The effect of prescribed daily dose frequency on patient medication compliance. Arch Intern Med 1990; *150*: 1881-4.

10 Ellard GA, Jenner PJ, Downs PA. An evaluation of the potential use of isoniazid, acetylisoniazid and isonicotinic acid for monitoring the self-administration of drugs. Br J Clin Pharmacol 1980; *10*: 369-81.

11 Eshelman FN, Fitzloff J. Effect of packaging on patient compliance with an antihypertensive medication. Curr Ther Res 1976; *20*: 215-8.

12 Eshelman FN, Fitzloff J, Troyer WG. Compliance rates for drug regimens in medical clinic patients. Clinical Trials J 1978; *15*: 3-15.

13 Evans L, Spelman M. The problem of non-compliance with drug therapy. Drug 1983; *25*: 63-76.

14 Feinstein AR. Clinical biostatistics. XXX Biostatistical problems in "compliance bias". Clin Pharm Ther 1974; *16*: 846-57.

15 Fitzgerald JD. The influence of the medication on compliance with a therapeutic regimen. In: Sackett DL, Haynes RB, eds. Compliance with therapeutic regimens. Baltimore: Johns Hopkins University Press 1976: 119-28.

16 Goldsmith CH. The effect of differing compliance distribution on the planning and statistical analysis of therapeutic trials. In: McMahon FG, ed. Principles and techniques of human research and therapeutics, vol. X: Lasagna L. Patient compliance. Mount Kisco: Futura 1976: 137-51.

17 Gordis L. Methodologic issues in the measurement of patient compliance. In Sackett DL, Haynes RB, eds. Compliance with therapeutic regimens. Baltimore: Johns Hopkins University Press 1976: 51-66.

18 Halperin M, Rogot E, Gurian J, Ederer F. Sample sizes for medical trials with special reference to long-term therapy. J Chron Dis 1968; *21*: 13-24

19 Haynes RB. A critical review of the "determinants" of patient compliance with therapeutic regimens. In: Sackett DL, Haynes RB, eds. Compliance with therapeutic regimens. Baltimore: Johns Hopkins University Press, 1976: 26-39.

20 Haynes RB. Strategies for improving compliance. A methodologic analysis and review. In: Sackett DL, Haynes RB, eds. Compliance with therapeutic regimens. Baltimore: Johns Hopkins University Press, 1976: 69-82.

21 Haynes RB, Sackett DL, Gibson ES et al. Improvement of medication compliance in uncontrolled hypertension. Lancet 1976; *i*: 1265-8.

22 Haynes RB, Sackett DL, Taylor DW, Robert RS, Johnson AL. Manipulation of the therapeutic regimen to improve compliance: conceptions and misconceptions. Clin Pharmacol Ther 1977; *22*: 125-30.

23 Hulka BS, Kuppler LL, Cassel JC, Efird RL, Burdette JA. Medication use and misuse: physician-patient discrepancies. J Chron Dis 1975; *28*: 7-21

24 Lima J, Nazarian L, Charney E, Lahti C. Compliance with short-term antimicrobial therapy: some techniques that help. Pediatrics 1976; *57*: 383-6.

25 Linkewich JA, Catalano RB, Flock HL. The effect of packaging and instruction on out-patient compliance with medication regimens. Drug Intelligence and Clinical Pharmacy 1974; *8*: 10-5.

26 Lowenthal DT, Briggs WA, Mutterperl R, Adelman B, Creditor MA. Patient compliance for antihypertensive medication: the usefulness of urine assays. Curr Ther Res 1976; *19*: 405-9.

27 Myers ED, Calvert EJ. The effect of forewarning on the occurrence of side-effects and discontinuance of medication in patients on dothiepin. J Int Med Res 1976; *4*: 237-40.

28 Peck CL, King NJ. Increasing patient compliance with prescriptions. JAMA 1982; *248*: 2874-7.

29 Pullar T, Kumar S, Tindall H, Feely M. Time to stop counting the tablets? Clin Pharmacol Ther 1989; *46*: 163-8.

30 Roth HP, Caron HS, Hsi BP. Measuring intake of a prescribed medication: a bottle count and a tracer technique compared. Clin Pharmacol Ther 1970; *11*: 228-337.

31 Rovelli M, Palmeri D, Vossler E et al. Non-compliance in organ transplant recipients. Transplantation Proceedings 1989; *21*: 833-4.

32 Rudd P, Marshall G, Taylor CB, Agras WS. Medication monitor/dispenser for pharmaceutical and compliance research. Clin Pharmacol Ther 1981; *29*: 278.

33 Rudd P, Ahmed S, Zachary V et al. Improved compliance measures: aplications in an ambulatory hypertensive drug trial. Clin Pharmacol Ther 1990; *48*: 676-85.

34 Sackett DL. The competing objectives of randomized trials. New Engl J Med 1980; *303*: 1059-60.

35 Sackett DL, Haynes RB, Gibson ES et al. Randomized trials of compliance-improving strategies in hypertension. In: MacMahon FG, ed. Principles and techniques of human research and therapeutics. vol. X: Lasagna L. Patient compliance. Mount Kisco: Futura 1976; 1-19.

36 Spriet A, Beiler D, Dechorgnat J, Simon P. Adherence of elderly patients to treatment with pentoxifyline. Clin Pharmacol Ther 1980; *27*: 1-8.

37 Spriet A, Dupin-Spriet T. a) Bonne pratique des essais cliniques des médicaments. Bâle: Karger, 1990; b) Good practice of clinical drug trials. Basel: Karger, 1992.

38 Stark JE, Ellard GA, Gammon PT, Fox W. The use of isoniazid as a marker to monitor the self-administration of medicaments. Br J Pharmac 1975; *2*: 355-8.

39 Weintraub M. Promoting patient compliance. Role of professionals, government, and the pharmaceutical industry. N Y State J Med 1975; *75*: 2263-6.

40 Weintraub M. Intelligent non-compliance and capricious non-compliance. In: McMahon FC, ed. Principles and techniques of human research and therapeutics vol. X: Lasagna L. Patient compliance. Mount Kisco: Futura: 1976; 39-47.

41 Weintraub M, Au WYW, Lasagna L. Compliance as a determinant of serum digoxin concentration. JAMA 1973; *224*: 481-5.

42 Witts DJ, Mulgirigama D, Turner P, Pare CMB. Some observations on patient compliance in an antidepressive trial. Postgrad Med J 1977; *53*: (suppl. 4), 136-8.

43 Yee RD, Hahn PM, Christensen RE. Medication monitor for ophthalmology. Amer J Ophthalmol 1974; *78*: 774-8.

12 - Case report forms

SUMMARY
The data for each participant in a clinical trial should be recorded on a form specially prepared for this purpose. Care should be taken to include all the information necessary to answer the questions asked in the protocol, but the record form should not be cluttered up with irrelevant or superfluous information.

The record form should contain information permitting identification of the subject, verification of group comparability, determination of treatment received prior to and during the study, patient compliance, assessment of outcome, adverse effects, the results of laboratory tests and the precise reasons for premature withdrawal from the trial.

Record forms should be clearly set out and neat, simple to use and check and, if possible, should facilitate automatic data processing by the use of pre-coded questions.

Several precautions are intended to make the case report forms practical for the users:

- design of re-usable standard pages,
- limitation of open questions,
- questions formulated so as to avoid all ambiguity,
- order of information adapted to data collection,
- memory aids for the investigator,
- clear and sufficiently spaced-out typing,
- verifications before and after printing,
- test runs,
- written instructions for filling out forms.

For each of the participants in a clinical trial, the necessary data must be recorded which will permit an analysis of the results. The data should be recorded in a case report form specially designed for the trial, in questionnaire form, so that all the relevant information for each patient will be recorded and available.

Designing the case report form, often bound in a patient book, is an important stage in the planning of a trial and should be given the necessary care and attention.

1. WHICH DATA SHOULD BE RECORDED ?

All of the items necessary for answering the questions asked by the trial protocol should be recorded (7, 9, 12).

The number of items must be restricted since there is no limit (15) to the amount of information that *might* be useful. Overly long report forms will tend to discourage the investigator (2) and are not often completely filled in. If the recording of a large number of items is possible, it is preferable to extend the baseline data rather than subsequent ones (10) since this will allow to define *a posteriori* subgroups of subjects with characteristics that may influence the response to the treatments compared (either favorably or unfavorably). It is always preferable to limit the information collected to that which is really expected to be useful for analyzing the results (3). This information generally coincides, in fact, with that which is required by regulations for the investigation of a new drug, and may be classified under several different headings (4).

1.1. Subject identification

To avoid confusing case-report forms and to allow a trial participant to be traced if necessary (in the case of an unforeseen result for example), the patient's *surname* and *first name* initials should appear on the report form.

For inpatients, recording the hospital number may also be useful.

1.2. Useful information for verifying group comparability

The following information is almost always necessary for verifying group comparability:
• Age and sex
• Body weight and sometimes height (because of their relationship with the effects of a given dose of drug).
• In some cases: the level of intellect (if the results are based, even partially, on the questioning of patients), ethnic groups, language comprehension or expression difficulties (if a standardized questionnaire is used or if the trial involves recording psychological items).
• Information concerning the illness treated, its severity, duration, particular clinical form (if applicable: symptomatic, etiologic, evolutive),

complications, concurrent disorders, and any recognized factors known to influence the prognosis of the illness under study during the time of the trial.

1.3 The treatment administered

Previous treatments and the reasons for their discontinuation, as well as any treatment begun or continued during the trial period should be recorded together with their duration, dosage, and the reason for their prescription.

The treatment under study should be noted using the treatment number assigned to the patient if the study is done "blind". The best technique is to prepare individually packaged vials, each with its own number printed on the label and duplicated on a detachable self-adhesive label that can be pasted on the patient's report form in a space set aside specifically for this purpose.

The amount of drug *actually taken* (rather than that stipulated in the protocol) should also be recorded together with any intercurrent changes and the reasons for the changes.

Whenever possible, compliance with therapy should be assessed on the basis of predetermined criteria.

1.4. Criteria of response

The therapeutic result is noted in compliance with assessment criteria stipulated.

1.5. Adverse events

Adverse events which may occur during a clinical trial are classified as minor or major. Recording of such events, their causal relationship with the test medication (12) and analysis of them are discussed in chapter 19.

1.6. Laboratory safety data

Adequate space should always be left in the case report forms for recording the results of laboratory tests stipulated in the protocol. Most commonly, a standardized page per visit is used for this purpose (14).

1.7. Uncompleted cases

For each subject who does not complete the anticipated trial period, it is indispensable to record the *reasons* for premature discontinuation of treatment. Ideally, this is done by filling out a pre-established check-list of all possible causes. This problem was dealt with in detail in chapter 10.

2. PRACTICAL DESIGN OF THE CASE REPORT FORMS

Preparation of case report forms requires considerable time. This work should not be given low priority after finalizing the protocol, but carried out in parallel and revised at each new version. Everything must be done to facilitate the collection and processing of data to prevent errors in filling out these forms and in entering data. The following propositions could serve to improve the presentation to satisfy these objectives (2, 8, 13, 14).

2.1. Use of standard pages

Standardized pages (or modules corresponding to parts of pages or to several pages) can be used in different trials (6). Their advantage is to avoid having to do repetitive work over again, by creating a new page for each trial. In addition, errors in development are avoided, since the standardized module has been validated (3) by usage. Standardized pages are usable for many data modules: demographics, medical histories, previous or concomitant treaments, adverse events, discontinuation of treatments or the end of the trial.

Other information can be recorded on "semi-standardized" pages: recording of laboratory test data and findings of the physical examination. The format and content is constant (wording of questions, number of characters, units), but some data can be added or rearranged.

Lastly, pages devoted to inclusion and exclusion criteria, to specific evaluations and to special investigations are most often specific. At best, for a few studies in the program of development of the same drug or of drugs in the same therapeutic class.

2.2. Limiting open questions

Blank fields intended to record descriptions or comments must be avoided. Descriptive text is difficult to process statistically and even to read and to interpret. Most information can be entered in numerical form or in the form of multiple choice questions and thus are precoded (5). In practice, open questions are only necessary for three types of information : morbidity (medical history, concomitant disorders), previous or concomitant treatments and adverse events (except those for which a specific checklist is prepared). These data will be processed after coding, preferentially by using a standard dictionary (WHO dictionary of adverse events, or COSTART, International Classification system of Diseases, the WHO drug reference list, etc.)

2.3. Improving the formulation of questions

If care is not taken, poorly formulated questions (16) or those difficult to answer may easily find their way into case report forms, for example:
- negative questions : "absence of ..." "no history of ..." or even double-

negative questions: "absence of an unauthorized drug: yes - no";

- relative questions: "improvement", "modification of treatment", with no precise reference to the preceding visit or to the initial visit, or even repeat relative questions, which are very difficult to answer, even if the time of reference has been defined;

- double questions joined by "and", "or" "and/or", "neither of the two";

- abbreviations which can mean different things to different participants: clinicians, nurses, statisticians, administrative personnel, even physicians practising different medical specialties;

- confusion between a checklist (each question must be answered) and multiple choice questions (a single question must be chosen out of several).

- numerical data for which the dimension of the fields is insufficient for some patients. In a certain number of cases, it is better to overestimate than to underestimate.

Special attention must be paid to translations of case report forms: opposite meanings in a specialized technical context commonly occur, even when the translation is performed by a competent translator.

2.4. Choosing the order of modules

The best choice is a controversial subject: strictly chronological order enables the filling out of information in the order in which it is available, thematic order (clinical evaluation of all visits, then laboratory data from all visits), facilitates comparison of data from one visit to another, permitting in particular detection of a "trend" for a specific variable.

In extended trials, chronological order is generally preferable since it enables information to be recorded at successive visits and to allow data processing as data are collected. In some cases, a synoptic presentation is nonetheless practical, in particular when it involves results obtained every hour in an intensive care unit, and recorded on sheets representing successive tests in parallel columns.

2.5. Memory aids

In a complex protocol, there are many opportunities to make mistakes or to forget to record information. Memory aids distributed to all critical areas of the case report forms can prevent these errors. They involve:

- steps in changes made in treatment (wash-out, decrease, fail-safe treatment, etc),

- dose titration guided by clinical results (including definition of rules for assignment of doses),

- appointment dates,

- information necessary to fill out the case report forms.

2.6. Typography

Each page should contain a separate and easily recognizable title and an area designated for recording the patient's identification.

Blocks of questions must be separated by appropriate spacing to assist in comprehension and filling out the form. One should not hesitate to "waste paper" in preparing the report from, spacing out the boxes to be filled in and in lining them up to facilitate verifying that they are properly filled in (figure 1). Boxes for recording alphanumeric information will preferably be squares at least 10 mm wide, without an upper horizontal line (open square) to avoid ambiguities in reading them.

Figure 1

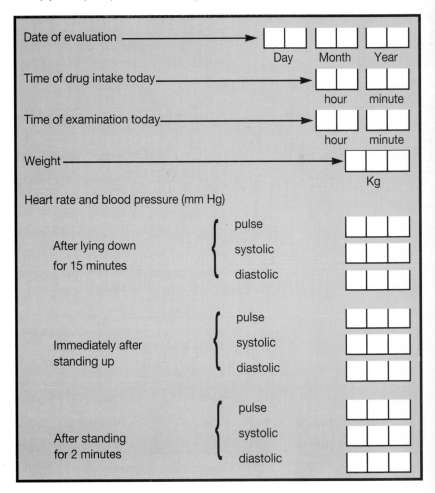

2.7 Verify the case report forms before they are printed

A quality control check list of the layout of the case report forms may be useful, by drawing attention to the following:

- the order of the information recorded,

- missing pages or forgotten modules,

- changes in page numbering during the drafting of successive versions,

- the size of spaces for recording answers,

- the content (a 100% correspondence between the case report forms and the protocol), memory aids, absence of obscure or ambiguous questions,

- the necessary step of performing a blank test run.

2.8. Quality of printing

Professionally-printed case report forms are easier and more pleasant to work with than home-made versions (2).

Many problems can be avoided by using good page design, high-performance word processors, good-quality self-duplicating paper (the last copy of which can still be read), securely bound copies preventing the loss of pages, and if possible individual number of a patient book printed on all pages.

2.9. Verification of printed copies

Incidents such as missing pages, pages bound upside down, printing faintly visible, paper color that does not conform, are sometimes discovered too late. Palliative measures taken afterwards only complicate data collection. In large trials, it is not possible to verify all pages in all copies but a few random checks are useful.

2.10. The test run

After the case report forms have been composed, it is a good practice to have them approved by the eventual users: monitors, clinical research assistants, investigators and data entry operations. It is also important to try and fill them out, even if they consist essentially of known standardized pages. From time to time it will be noted during this phase that considering the context, the formulation of some questions is not appropriate. One or more case report forms should be filled out: at least with fabricated data, and by at least one of the investigators. Poorly-formulated or ambiguous questions are often discovered during this phase.

3. DOCUMENTS FOR SELF-EVALUATION

If some of the information is to be recorded by the patient himself, properly identifiable detachable pages should be prepared and provision should be made for inserting them into the record book without the risk of loss. If information has to be recorded daily by an outpatient, he should be given a special notebook containing a very simple questionnaire and all the necessary explanations.

The patient should be carefully instructed as to how to record data correctly and equal care should be taken in ensuring that he has done so (7).

4. INSTRUCTIONS FOR FILLING IN PATIENT REPORT FORMS

A special page 1 instruction page for filling out the report forms should be planned containing the following:

- rules for using self-duplicating paper:

"you are going to fill out a case report form in triplicate to be used in a clinical trial. We ask that you do so using <u>a black ball-point pen</u> so that copies are clearly legible, and by reinserting the protective cardboard dividers between each set of pages to avoid accidentally marking subsequent pages".

- general rules to answer questions:

"we wish to call your attention to the fact that <u>all questions must be answered</u> either with the information asked for or by marking a slanted line when the information does not exist". Whenever it is necessary to write out a descriptive text (open questions) it is important for it to be clearly legible (if possible, <u>print</u> answers).

- rules for filling in boxes:

Numerical values should be correctly entered in each square starting at the right if no decimal point is marked, or in relation to a printed decimal point.

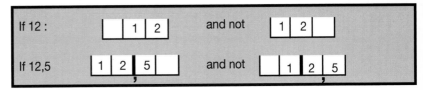

- rules for correction of erroneous data:

"If you have to make a correction, we ask you to please do the following :
• cross out the answer with a single line, allowing the erroneous information to be still legible,
• write the date the correction was made,
• sign your name".

Case report forms are important for recording reliable data. A minimum number of precautions makes it possible to obtain good-quality documents. Even in studies using remote data entry systems via computer terminals, a paper copy generally is necessary for a large part of the data, and in any case the same rules apply to the preparation of screens for entering data.

References

1 Altman DG. Statistics and ethics in medical research. Collecting and screening data Br Med J 1980; *281*: 1399-401.

2 Bennett AE, Ritchie K. Questionnaires in medicine. Oxford: University Press 1975.

3 Bernd Cl. Clinical case report form design. A key to clinical trials success. Drug Information Journal 1984; *18*: 3-8.

4 Burke WE. Buday PV. Patients report forms: their design and use in drug evaluation. Curr Ther Res 1965; *7*: 422-434.

5 Feinstein AR. Taxonorics. II. Formats and coding systems for data processing. Arch Intern Med 1970; *126*: 1053-67.

6 Grady F. Designing the report form. In: Good CS, Clarke C, eds. The principle and practice of clinical trials. Edinburgh: Churchill Livingstone 1976: 60-74.

7 Hamilton M. Planning of team research. Br Vet J 1967; *123*: 375-82.

8 Leferrière N, Tenaillon A, Saltiel JC et al. Le questionnaire médical. Principes - construction et évaluation - applications. Paris: INSERM, 1978.

9 Leighton CC. Design and use of clinical case report forms. In: McMahon FG, ed. Principles and techniques of human research and therapeutics, vol. IV: Importance of experimental design and bio-statistics. Mount Kisco: Futura, 1974.

10 Peto R, Pike MC, Armitage P et al. Design and analysis of randomized clinical trials requiring prolonged observation of each patient. II Analysis and examples. Br J Cancer 1977; *35*: 1-39.

11 Skegg DCG, Doll R. The case for recording events in clinical trials. Br Med J 1977; *2*: 1523-4.

12 Spilker B, Schoenfelder J. Data collection forms in clinical trials. New York: Raven Press, 1991.

13 Spriet A, Dupin-Spriet T. How to improve case report forms. In: Ferran J, Lahuerta Dal Re J, Lardinois R, eds. Communication in pharmaceutical medicine: a challenge for 1992. Barcelona: Prous Science Publishers, 1991: 85-8.

14 Spriet A, Dupin-Spriet T. a) Réalisation d'un cahier d'observation. In: Bonne pratique des essais cliniques des médicaments. Bâle: Karger, 1990: 55-63. b) Designing the case report forms. In: Good practice of clinical drug trials. Basel: Karger, 1992: 57-65.

15 Weintraub M. Recording events in clinical trials. Br Med J 1978; *1*: 581.

16 Wright R, Haybittle J. Design of forms for clinical trials. (a) Br Med J 1979; *2*: 529-30. (b) Br Med J 1979; *2*: 590-2. (c) Br Med J 1979; *2*: 650-2.

13 - Multicenter trials

SUMMARY
Clinical trials performed simultaneously by several investigators using the same protocol with a view to pooling the data for analysis, permit broad recruitment of patients.

Several requirements must be met in a multicenter trial. The participating centers must be chosen to be comparable with regard to their equipment, staff and the type of patient seen. The standardization of the methods used for measuring study parameters is for reducing "intercenter" variability to the level that might be expected by random variation alone, and standardized follow-up.

Coordination is necessary to control the initiation and progress of the trial and the verification and analysis of the data.

The analysis of the results should include a study of the comparability of the participating centers (with regard to recruitment and results), the "center" factor and possible "center by treatment" interaction.

A multicenter trial (10) is a clinical trial conducted simultaneously by several investigators working in different institutions but using the same protocol, identical methods in order to pool the data collected and analyze them together.

A multicenter trial may range from a small trial with two or three investigators who collect a relatively small number of cases in the space of a few months to a much larger operation in which thousands of patients are enlisted by dozens of institutions over a period of several years.

The problems of standardization and coordination are basically the same regardless of the size of the trial, but the greater the number of participants and the more complex the trial, the more difficult those problems are to overcome.

On the other hand, it is incorrect to form a "multicenter trial" by grouping together the results of studies planned to be separate, even conducted with an identical protocol. This approach can only be presented in the context of a *meta-analysis*. It is even more questionable to only group together selected studies or centers (18).

1. A MAJOR ADVANTAGE OF MULTICENTER TRIALS : A LARGER AND MORE REPRESENTATIVE PATIENT SAMPLE

If we wish to conduct a clinical trial to study a rare disorder or a very restrictively-defined patient population, recruitment of enough appropriate patients in a single center within a reasonable period of time is often impossible. By having several physicians (or hospitals) participate in a study, not only will patient accrual be increased but these patients will also be more "representative" of the entire patient population owing to the somewhat different local population characteristics of each center.

Consequently, the generalization of the results will be more valid.

An important question involves the choice between few centers recruiting many patients or many centers recruiting few patients. The answer is obvious for rare illnesses where it is mandatory to multiply the number of centers so that recruitment does not "go on forever" and to observe that quality suffers.

For commonly-occurring illnesses, it is generally easier to standardize, to follow and to motivate a small number of centers. The only advantage of having many "small" centers (apart from marketing considerations) is perhaps a better representativity.

Unless it is absolutely impossible to do so, the extreme situation of having one case per center should be avoided because it does not enable differentiating between a center-related effect and one related to the treatments.

2. SPECIAL REQUIREMENTS FOR MULTICENTER TRIALS

2.1. Comparability of participating institutions

Data collected from several centers cannot be analyzed together unless the centers themselves are comparable from the viewpoint of equipment, staff and types of patients recruited (5). It is therefore indispensable to conduct a systematic survey of organization and function of each center before commencing the trial.

2.1.1. Equipment

If a laboratory test or investigation is to be used as an assessment criterion in a multicenter trial, the organizers must be certain that the test can be performed under the same conditions and that its results are equally reliable in each center. This requires that equipment (spirometers, treadmills, etc.) and methods, including assay methods, be standardized. Samples can be sent to a single laboratory, either to check the results from each individual laboratory, or better still, to carry out the most important tests, in particular, the one chosen as the principal criterion of efficacy.

2.1.2. Staff

The number of staff members, their availability and experience in conducting clinical trials should be similar from one center to another.

2.1.3. Recruitment

The number of patients in each center should not be too dissimilar, nor should the patient population be too heterogeneous with regard to demographic, pathologic and other characteristics. Besides, centers producing few cases are often those where data quality is mediocre (17).

2.2. A common protocol

If the data from several centers are to be analyzed together, they must obviously have been obtained using identical methodology. A certain degree of "inter-center" variability may of course be taken into account in the analysis, but this variation should reflect no more than sampling fluctuations.

Patient enlistment, methods for assessing the results must all be specified.

Any differences in the interpretation of the protocol from one center to another may result in a lack of homogeneity. A protocol intended for multicenter use must therefore be much more detailed than one intended for use by a single investigator. The protocol or its appendices or separate procedures (operation manual) should attempt to foresee all questions which may arise (6). It is desirable that the protocol be discussed during the planning stage with at least some investigators, especially if it is innovative and original in its content. Furthermore, within each institution, it is a very useful habit to have a detailed discussion with the *entire staff involved in the trial*, notably when the trial is being set up.

2.3. Coordinating the trial

In all but the smallest multicenter trials, a coordinating group made up of specialists should be set up. The members of such a group should meet frequently and they should be able to devote the necessary time to directing and controlling the way the trial is set up and conducted.

2.3.1. Composition of the coordinating group

The composition of the coordinating group will vary depending on the nature of the trial but generally includes a clinician, a statistician, a person who is responsible for on-site trial monitoring, and possibly a pharmacologist and one or more specialists in different fields involved in the trial. The coordinating center should have adequate secretarial facilities, data processing equipment and should be readily contactable by telephone.

In large multicenter trials, several committees might be required (4) including:
- a coordinating center,
- a steering committee,
- an advisory board of experts,
- an ethics committee,
- a committee to monitor adverse events.

2.3.2. Role of the coordinating group

The role of the coordinating group may vary from one trial to another but it may involve the following functions (5, 7, 8, 11, 12, 14) :
- designing and planning a protocol draft,
- discussing the protocol with all interested parties,
- organizing pre-trial meetings,
- writing up the final protocol,
- motivating the investigators once the initial period of enthusiasm is over (14).

It is important to take into account the factors that contribute to motivating the investigators. Some of the most important factors include :

- a legitimate desire for scientific recognition which can be satisfied by fair distribution of co-authorship of publications, sometimes by preparing several manuscripts on special aspects. Lists of participants may also be published and the participants may acquire the rights to claim membership to a cooperative group if the latter becomes permanent;

- allocation of funds which should be equitably distributed among the participants at all levels, according to the work done;

- the advantages of belonging to a working party which may meet, within the framework of the trial or even in another context, to foster the exchange of ideas and experiences between specialists in different fields;

- discussion of the randomization procedure, the packaging of drugs used in the trial, and the case report forms used,

- informing the investigators about how the trial is progressing, the incidents that may have occurred, the difficulties encountered or the errors committed. It is a good idea, for example, to organize intermediate meetings, preferably in a different center each time, so that all the participants can keep abreast of what is being done in centers other than their own,

- discussion of protocol amendments considered necessary during the course of the trial,

- decisions concerning imperfect data (protocol violations or incomplete case reports) if possible according to criteria written in advance in the protocol or in the operating procedures,

- in extreme case, exclusion of one of the participating centers if it becomes apparent that the data from this center is consistently unreliable,

• replacing a center that is unable or unwilling to continue participating in a trial.

Sometimes there is confusion on the role of the coodinating committees, since in some trials the same agency is in charge both of coordination and of subcontracting certain tasks (on-site monitoring, verification of data, analyses of results, etc...)

3. SPECIFIC DIFFICULTIES IN INTERNATIONAL TRIALS (3, 15, 16)

When a very large-scale trial is undertaken in several countries, additional difficulties may arise owing to differences in many factors :

- differences in language, in particular for patient questionnaires and labelling of test drugs,
- certain concepts of disease and treatment,
- equipment used for investigations,
- drug dosages (need for a consensus on dosage of the comparator),
- content and time of meals,
- ethnic differences (metabolism and stature)...

Translations of the protocol will be required but there must be a reference version in a language understood by all the participants.

4. THE FEASIBILITY PILOT TRIAL

For trials intended to continue for several years and to enroll a very large number of patients, it is desirable to request that each center conduct a pilot trial involving a few cases. This will provide information about (9):

• expected patient accrual in each center,

• the feasibility of the study (the protocol may not be realistic),

• the quality of data collected, making it possible to determine the errors or omissions to be avoided,

• the comparability of centers with regard to the patients selected and the manner in which the data is collected,

• patient acceptability and potential side-effects of the treatments studied,

• the variability of the results, which may make it possible to calculate the number of subjects needed to achieve a given type 2 error for the comparison (or conversely, to calculate the power of the tests used to compare groups of a given size),

• possibly, factors which have a strong influence on the results and which must be taken into account in a stratification.

Feasibility pilot studies, by their very nature, are necessarily limited to short observation periods. In a trial involving preventive treatment where follow-up and evaluation may last for several years, a pilot study can be conducted only for early evaluations, which is still better than nothing!

A ticklish question is whether to include the results of a pilot study in the final analysis. This is acceptable *provided that no changes have been made in the protocol following the pilot study. In fact, a protocol is seldom maintained unchanged after a pilot study since its purpose is to detect and rectify weak points and a protocol is never perfect...* The investigators may have to "learn" an unfamiliar measurement procedure and this may disqualify pilot study data from inclusion in the overall report.

5. ANALYSIS OF THE RESULTS

Several problems specific to multicenter trials must be considered :

5.1. The "center" factor

Incorporation of the *"center" factor* into the analysis improves the power of comparison of treatments. This makes it possible to deduce the *variability between centers* from the *residual variability* and thus to make detection of differences between treatments more sensitive. This method enables taking into account only those centers which have contributed at least one case per treatment. If sample sizes in some centers are too small, it may be useful to pool them into a "big center".

5.2. Interaction

Furthermore, it is important to verify if the difference between treatments vary outside random fluctuations across all centers. If major differences exist, they can be demonstrated by a significant result in a test of interaction *"treatment per center"*. The cause should then be sought (13).

5.2.1. Causes

• Differences in patient features from one center to another:

The influence of these characteristics is *confounded* with the influence of the centre. If there is a major difference, it can result in limiting extrapolation of the results to some categories of subjects.

• An abnormal frequency of protocol violations, losses to follow-up or non-compliers in one or more centers, which may reflect poor adherence to the protocol or insufficient motivation of investigators in these centers.

• "Outlyer" center (2), possibly due to a small number of doubtful cases.

Doubtful results issuing from a centre may decrease credibility concerning these data and this may be discussed in the final interpretation of results. However, it is not permissible to exclude them (as this might lead to abuse), except in an appendix to the main analysis.

• Real variations of differences between treatments according to centers (restricting the generalization of results to any medical team).

5.2.2. Interpretation

In practice, such a significant "treatment per center" interaction is *embarassing in two cases*: if the difference observed in the overall results comes from a single center, or if there is a *"cross-over"* interaction, with differences between treatments in opposite directions from different centers (one treatment better than the other in some centers, and the opposite in other centers). In this case, one should also consider the number of centers and the proportion of centers contradictory to global analysis: the more numerous, the more "embarassing". If a satisfactory explanation is not found, an analysis with and without the "abnormal" center can be presented (analysis N-1).

It is necessary to take into account the *number of patients* recruited by each center.

Ideally, each centre should provide a similar number of patients. Although it is not ideal, differences of sample-sizes are frequent between centers. In case of a cross-over interaction, if the "contradictory" centers give a small contribution to the sample size, it is less embarassing than if their recruitment is important. Sometimes, the question of weighted analyses should be raised: should equal weights be given to individual cases or to individual centers? In the first case, more importance is given to centers with important enrollment, in the second case more importance is given to cases from centers with poor recruitment.

5.3. Analysis of results center by center

Separate analysis of results from each center is dangerous (1). By definition, the number of patients available in an isolated center is insufficient to allow drawing conclusions, and publication of only "positive" centers overestimates the difference. Nonetheless, separate analyses are sometimes required by government agencies as a descriptive measure, to be able to evaluate the homogeneity of results.

Such analyses can also be useful for the interpretation of a center by investigator interaction.

References

1 Anonymous. Reporting of single-centre evidence from multi-centre therapeutic trials. Pharmaceutical Medicine 1988; *2*: 312-3.

2 Canner PL, Huang YB, Meinert CL. On the detection of outlier clinics in medical and surgical trials. I. Practical considerations. Controlled Clinical Trials 1981; *2*: 231-41.

3 Dick P, Angst J, Battegay R et al. Problèmes des essais thérapeutiques multicentriques (à propos d'une tentative de collaboration des 5 cliniques psychiatriques universitaires suisses). Proc. IVth World Conf Psychiatry Madrid, Sept 1966. Intern Conf Series No.150. Amsterdam: Excerpta Medica Foundation, 1968; 823-5.

4 Ederer F. Practical problems in collaborative clinical trials. Amer J Epidemiol 1975; *102*: 111-8.

5 Finkel MJ. Responsibilities of clinical monitors and clinical investigators. Presented at the Associates of Clinical Pharmacology Meeting. San Francisco, California, March 20, 1980.

6 Greenberg BG. Conduct of cooperative field and clinical trials. The American Statistician 1959; *13*: 18-28.

7 Hamilton M. Planning of team research. Br Vet J 1967; *123*: 375-82.

8 Klimt CR, Meinert CL. The design and methods of cooperative therapeutic trials with examples from a study on diabetes. Intern Encycl Pharmacol Therap Clinical Pharmacology. Lasagna L, ed. 1976, *Vol.1*, chap. 19, 341-73.

9 Mason BJ. Organization of a multi-centre trial. Geront Clin 1974; *16*: 105-9.

10 Meinert CL. Toward more definitive clinical trials. Controlled Clinical Trials 1980; *1*: 249-61.

11 Meinert CL. Organization of multicenter clinical trials. Controlled Clinical Trials 1981; *1*: 05-12.

12 Mowery R, Williams OD. Aspect of clinic monitoring in large scale multiclinic trials. Clin Pharmacol Ther 1979; *25*: 717-9.

13 Overall JE. General linear model analysis of variance. In: Levine J, ed. Coordinating clinical trials in psychopharmacology. Rockville MD: NIMH, 1979; 63-85.

14 Sherry S. Trial and error, questions and answers. In: Thrombosis, pathogenesis and clinical trials. Stuttgart: Schattauer Verlag, 1973: 263-70.

15 Spilker B. National versus multinational clinical trials. Drug News and Perspectives 1990; *4*: 469-79.

16 Spriet A. Les essais multicentriques internationaux. Méd Hyg 1990; *48*: 1286-7.

17 Sylvester RJ, Pinedo HM, De Pauw M et al. Quality of institutional participation in multicenter clinical trials. New Engl J Med 1981; *305*: 852-8.

18 Temple R. Effective design of clinical studies. Drug Information Journal 1986; *20*: 127-33.

14 - Imperfect data analysis

SUMMARY   *Trial planning should prevent errors, but imperfections are unavoidable. Transparency is necessary (listing and description of imperfections as well as rules to deal with imperfect data should be given in the trial report). Decisions on data should be made independent of the results: written rules, and independent and blind decisions are necessary.*

Between purism and laxism, realistic rules are often acceptable. Rules are proposed for the most frequent situations: missing data, outliers, cases of protocol violations, treatment discontinuations, poor compliance, and losses to follow-up.

Intent-to-treat analysis avoids biased post hoc exclusions, but a few exceptions are acceptable in extreme cases.

"Sensitivity analysis" enables testing the robustness of results to some decisions on data.

Perfect data from a clinical trial are obtained when all patients selected are randomized, satisfy all inclusion-exclusion criteria, receive 100% of the medication doses, undergo all desired evaluations within the exact calendar and are followed up to the planned date. This perfection is exceptional.

Although trial planners must devote all possible efforts to developing a realistic design, and to closely monitoring its execution, this will only make errors rarer, and never eradicate them completely.

Analysis of data has to take into account imperfections, not in an effort to mask or cover them up, but to analyze their influence on the final report.

Nevertheless, the possibility of using incomplete and flawed data should not be overemphasized to the investigator, otherwise he will feel encouraged to relax his efforts of rigor and thoroughness.

The rules developed here are supposed to be applied to honest (non-fraudulent) data cleaned from entry transcription errors. We suggest several rules applicable for all situations, and examples of specific statements for a number of abnormalities (missing values, outliers, protocol violations, treatment discontinuations, and losses to follow-up).

1. GENERAL RULES

Imperfect data impose various decisions concerning likelihood, evaluability, replacement scores, and analytical methods. Such decisions are "neutral" and can influence the trial outcome and conclusions. Therefore, careful precautions must be taken.

1.1. Transparency of imperfections and of decisions

The first rule is to describe in study reports, case by case or with tabulations, all imperfections so that the reader may weigh the results against his own credibility scale. It is typically a separate chapter in the final study report. The following imperfections should be listed and detailed:

- Missing data,
- Outliers,
- Protocol violations,
- Noncompliers,
- Losses to follow-up,
- Treatment discontinuations.

In addition, rules for using those data should be given clearly, including who made the decision, when it was made (before, during, and after data clearing procedures), and whether data were screened blindly of the randomized treatment.

1.2. A realistic attitude

The purist methodologist simply assumes that the trial should be designed so that it will be possible to collect complete data and only data that conform and are perfectly executed.

Faced with many imperfections, he will simply refuse to look at the results. If he finally admits reluctantly that a few unavoidable problems occurred, he will recommend extreme, rigorous attitudes, which can hardly result in any conclusions from the data.

The laxist methodologist is very flexible in his design, anticipating th rigid rules will not be followed. He will accept sloppy data and witho restriction, arrange, estimate, replace and exclude some data to mal them fit a statistical model.

He then draws unrestricted conclusions. If these conclusions are fals he will assign them to the random error he is "right" to make once in while from the statistical theory of tests.

In between, the realist will be careful in design and execution, he w refuse to draw conclusions from poor quality data, but will app acceptable rules to imperfections, considering the complexity in case-b case situations: frequency of abnormalities, influence on outcome clinical context, foreseeable problems, unbiased decisions, ar imperfections whether balanced or not by treatment groups. In th paper, we will try to adopt this intermediate attitude.

1.3. Rules formulated in advance

Rules should be chosen as early as possible. Most of them can k anticipated in the design phase and some are to be incorporated into th study protocol. Sometimes, one or more published references can k quoted or listed in an appendix.

Nevertheless, it is counterproductive to reveal too many details in th study protocol on how to arrange imperfect data: it gives som investigators a false impression that sloppiness has no consequence and is always amendable without any problems! Therefore, rules are be detailed in an appendix or in a separate standard procedure, containir results of internal consensus, established in advance, and available to th team of the data manager and the biometrician working in the clinic trials program. The procedure is also available for audit and inspection case it is contested. This procedure defines who is responsible fc decisions on data, describes documents necessary for this evaluatio lists most important cases and standard acceptable rules, requires written document describing decisions, and controls incorporation c items into the final report.

1.4. Reproducibility

If possible, decisions of the same nature for all cases in the same tri should be made simultaneously, preferably in a single session or at lea in a few sessions, to avoid inconsistencies.

1.5. Independence

Often, some particular cases could not have been anticipatec unforeseeable rules must be devised. If critical choices on particula cases, with possible significant influence on the results, have to be made, they should preferably be taken by someone independent of the trial: a consultant or a committee.

1.6. "Blindness" of patient therapy

Decisions will be less biased if they are made *blindly* by persons unaware of the patient's treatment. This is sometimes extremely difficult to realize, particularly if the treatments were not blind to the investigators. In that case, blinded case reports and data listing have to be prepared for the independent data reviewers.

1.7. Blindness of the trial outcome

If post hoc decisions happen to be necessary they should be taken before any preliminary statistical analyses give an idea of the results and can therefore influence choices.

1.8. Limited loss of information

Imperfect data should be used as much as possible since exclusion of data from analyses decreases power and can be responsible for biases.

1.9. Intention to treat analyses or evaluable cases

In theory, all patients randomized should be present in the main analysis. Exclusion of non-evaluable cases makes groups no longer comparable since they were not withdrawn from analyses at random.

In many clinical situations this position is valid: the purpose of the trial is then to evaluate the effect of *deciding to prescribe* a treatment whether or not it is administered to the right patients. In practice, if the new treatment is adopted, it will be prescribed under the same conditions. Nevertheless, in some cases, exclusion from analysis of a small number of cases where diagnosis is not confirmed from data collected before enrollment is acceptable if such cases are rare, balanced and if diagnostic confirmation is made blindly (13).

Apart from this extreme case, the following rules can be proposed:

- a full description of all entry violations is given in the study report by type of violation and by arm of the study (numbers and baseline characteristics).

- a first "attenuated" intention-to-treat analysis is performed maintaining all doubtful or erroneous diagnoses, but excluding only patients who after randomization received *no dose* of the therapy or had *no evaluation* after at least one dose of therapy. The full description of these rules is given in the study report.

- If a second analysis is performed with post hoc exclusions (decided independently and blindly), it is exploratory and complements the main analysis.

1.10. Sensitivity analysis

An affective compromise to make when there are good reasons to hesitate between two methods which can bias the results in opposite directions is to do a sensitivity analysis. Often it takes the form of an intention-to-treat analysis compared to an analysis per protocol (perfect conformity to protocol).

Both analyses are done and their results compared. If they go approximately in the same direction, the results are robust with respect to assumptions implied by the rules. In the opposite case, an explanation has to be found, justified, and discussed. Nevertheless, sensitivity analysis should not be multiplied with different types of imperfections, otherwise interpretation can be obscured.

2. MISSING VALUES

Occasionally, some information is unavailable or lost. The reason is not always sloppiness on the part of the investigator: ruined blood samples, temporary technical failure of a device for measurement, information not remembered by the patient, lost documents and so forth. Too many missing data make the trial unusable, but a few do not significantly alter the results. There are, therefore, two questions to answer :

• What does "too many" mean ?

• How can results be analyzed with a few missing data ?

2.1. Are there too many missing data ?

In general, the tolerable number of missing data is that which is only a fraction of the information which would significantly change the outcome, were all missing data masking an effect in opposite direction.

In the case of a controlled clinical trial comparing two treatments, an approach to detect whether this level is reached would be, in some cases, to perform a sensitivity analysis with two opposite assumptions: all missing scores are favorable for one treatment, and unfavorable for the other, and vice-versa.

2.2. Can missing data be replaced ?

Some statistical models enable analysis with incomplete data. They assume that presence or absence of information cannot be linked to a treatment effect, and that it will not influence the results. If these conditions are not fulfilled, missing data should be replaced by a replacement score. Estimation from other cases is usually unsatisfactory.

Estimation for other variables of the same individual is acceptable if the variables are well-correlated or almost redundant with the missing one. This condition should, therefore, be checked.

It is simpler and more reasonable to simply replace a missing value from one case by the preceding value (in time) from the same individual. This is possible in repeated measurement trials with data missing from one visit but present at the preceding visit.

In some particular cases, missing values are known to be extreme values (in particular in laboratory tests where results would have been below or above limits of detection). Those cases should be considered outliers with true extreme values (cf. below).

3. OUTLIERS

Extreme values from one variable can occur. After the necessary inquiry from source-documents and from the investigator's memory, they can be true, false or doubtful.

• A surely "false" value can come from a mistake in transcription, a device failure, or a technical error. The value is without a doubt impossible (subject 20 feet tall, Natremia 240 meq, Hamilton Depression Score 200), but the true value cannot be found. We suggest considering them missing values.

• "True" extreme values occur when a result is clearly outside of the usual range for the selected population, but has been verified : an extremely high number of onsets of a recurrent disease, unlimited exercise test, very slow spontaneous heart rate, or extremely high levels of cholesterol. Extreme unknown values outside the measurable range may fall in the same category. In all those cases, the true values should be analyzed, but may not fit the planned statistical analysis. In particular, they might require changing an initially planned parametric method for a non-parametric one. If this solution is not applicable (sophisticated non parametric methods do not exist for all possible study designs), "Winsorization" can be used. The extreme value is replaced by the one immediately following it by values in decreasing order (3, 5).

• Doubtful extreme values are the most delicate cases. They will fall within either of the preceding categories depending on arbitrary decisions. Therefore, they must be screened one by one, if possible by independent reviewers, blindly of the therapies, with a uniform rule, and before the first statistical analysis. Their being extreme has to follow clinical judgments and not only statistical distribution screening from the data of the trial itself. In particular, use of tests for outliers to systematically reject the largest or the smallest value for a variable is not recommended. Statistical tests for detection of outliers are often of no great use since they assume normal distributions while true outlying values are likely to occur in skewed distributions (5). Deviations from the mean by 4 or 5 standard deviations are rare but not impossible. The method is acceptable to detect extreme values but not to exclude unlikely values (1).

4. PROTOCOL VIOLATIONS

Complex protocols are hard to follow without encountering any problems. Minor deviations and even some major violations will occur. If the frequency of violations is such that they can jeopardize reasonable conclusions, data will be useful only to plan a better further study! In other cases, deviations have to be taken into account (15).

There are many causes of protocol violations.

- Some come from the protocol: ambiguities, uncompleteness, complexities, or obscure items might not become apparent until late in the execution of the trial.

- The investigator can be the cause: he forgot, overlooked the importance of details, or was too busy to conduct the trial correctly.

- The patients might bear some responsibility: they forgot appointments, lost self-monitoring forms, took unauthorized medications, or did not mention previous diseases in their history.

- Technical failures (erroneous laboratory test) can lead to erroneous inclusions or unwarranted adjustment of therapy.

The consequences of protocol violations and the necessary decisions vary from case to case (15). We will classify them by types of violations.

4.1. Non-inclusion of an eligible case (pre-randomization)

This is not really a protocol violation. The consequences can be : decreased recruitment, prolongation of inclusion period, and selective differentiation of selected cases which can restrict generalization of results, but not bias the results. Nevertheless, if nonincluded cases are entered in an entry log, it can be useful to know to which population the results can be generalized and to interpret discordant results from other trials by different patient selections (12).

4.2. Inclusion of noneligible cases

This violation is much more serious and the consequences are different according to the many subtypes:

4.2.1. Violation of inclusion criteria

Violations of inclusion criteria include :

• Completely erroneous diagnoses (a bad indication or even a contraindication for one of the compared treatments). This can happen if a diagnostic test (ECG, X-ray) performed before inclusion had an erroneous interpretation and was corrected later. Exclusion from analysis of a few clearly erroneous diagnoses is conceivable if eligibility criteria are unambiguous and unchallengeable (14).

• Unconfirmed diagnoses based on data available after inclusion. This case has to be subdivided into cases where data (i.e. blood sample) was collected *before* treatment (i.e. treatment of septicemia started before blood culture results are available), or *after* it (acute myocardial infarction before typical ECG and increased enzyme levels are observed). In the latter case one should consider whether treatment could influence the results of those tests or not (7).

• In all other cases, posthoc exclusion is not recommended, particularly if their proportion is high. Subgroup analysis of perfectly eligible patients can be given as subsidiary analysis (8). These cases comprise:

- doubtful diagnoses, for which key data are missing, or

- cases which are too mild or too serious, are clearly outside the operational range of severity scores.

4.2.2. Violation of exclusion criteria

Consequences are different according to the reason for exclusion:

• Evaluability exclusion: aimed at avoiding inclusion of cases with anticipated difficulty in evaluation (illiterate patients given reading material, arthrosic subjects undergoing treadmill test, arrhythmia patients with ambulatory blood pressure measurement). If such cases are erroneously included, exclusion from analyses, provided they are exceptional, is tolerable : if there is a partial evaluation, then the case falls in the category of missing-data.

• Follow-up clauses: if the exclusion criteria aimed at preventing losses to follow-up (unstable or uncooperative patients, travellers, etc...). In case of violations, one should distinguish those actually lost to follow-up and those who actually came back to the planned visits. Only the former should be treated as losses to follow-up.

• Safety exclusion: if the exclusion was motivated by some potential danger (contra-indication to one of the treatments or one of the procedures of the trial), the nonexcluded patients might or might not have developed the dangerous reaction. They should be included in the :

- efficacy and safety analysis if no serious reaction happened, or

- at least safety analysis if a serious reaction happened early and prevented the collection of any efficacy data.

4.3. Error in allocation

Sometimes treatments are not administered to successive patients according to the order given by a randomization list. In theory, patients should be analyzed in the group they should have belonged to, had the randomization order been complied with. Although this purist rule is acceptable for some efficacy analysis, it is not tolerable for safety reports. In practice, the consequences of this violation are different in blinded and unblinded trials.

4.3.1. Double-blind trials

In double-blind trials, the randomization list is prepared in advance and used to label the drug units. If in isolated cases, one drug unit was given by permuting two numbers and if we are sure that the investigator did not recognize the content (breaking the blindness), we would accept keeping the patient in the group whose treatment he actually received, assuming that the error was random and could only upset the balance within one block. The violation should, of course, be mentioned in the report.

If, on the contrary, allocation is systematically mixed up in a trial (or in one center of a multicenter trial), there is some suspicion that someone in the investigator's staff actually tried to recognize the drug and tried to target indications. In that case, any efficacy analysis is hopeless. Results of individual cases can be listed, and safety could be analyzed by the groups of the actual treatment.

If it were only a naive rerandomization mix-up by someone on the investigator's staff ignoring the basic methodological rules, and if breaking the blindness can be excluded, some sensitivity analysis (according to planned randomization and according to actual treatment) can be proposed (2). In any event, unbalanced groups should be analyzed with discussion of their influence on the results.

4.3.2. Unblinded trials

In the case of unblinded trials with allocation envelopes, systematic violations of the randomization order raises the suspicion of unblinded patient selection. This occurs when one envelope is opened in advance for the next patient. This is no longer a true randomization and selection bias is suspected. Subjects can be selected knowing the treatment they will receive! An unbalanced group can become evident. This case is hopeless (except for safety analysis of the new treatment). For this reason, allocation using plain envelopes (without possible control of opening time), should be replaced as often as possible by the surer blind allocation (telephone, fax or remote data entry).

4.4. Timing errors

Planned visits or tests are occasionally done outside the planned margin of tolerance for dates or times. Occasionally, the whole program of visits is shifted. There is no better solution than to take available values which are as close as possible to the planned times (2). A table of replacement times will be given in the violations chapter of the report.

4.5. Assessment errors

Assessment errors can happen when the investigator does not use the planned method for measuring the main criteria (he uses a more convenient or cheaper one, or the planned device had a technical failure, etc.). In such cases, an intention to treat analysis is done, with a discussion of the influence of the change on the results.

4.6 Dosing errors

Dosing errors are particularly worrisome in trials with dose adjustments done according to clinical outcome. Doses must be increased or decreased by predetermined steps if some efficacy variable (blood pressure, rating scale, laboratory test) reached a given threshold.
Unfortunately, in some patients the dose was not adjusted when it should have been, or it was increased or decreased too fast. This protocol violation will, of course, be described in the study report. The analysis may raise special problems. If the trial was intended to determine an optimal dosage, it may be useful to analyze these violations as a separate subgroup (exploratory analysis). Otherwise the intention-to-treat principle will be applied. In any case, safety analyses will relate adverse events to the dose actually given.

4.7. Broken blindness

In double blind trials, bias is possible if the nature of the treatment is guessed before final assessment of each case. This can occur for many reasons. The randomization list was not hidden in a safe place from staff responsible for collecting or correcting data, too many code envelopes were opened in cases of an emergency or without a good reason (4), the drugs appearance were initially distinguishable or gradually became distinguishable (i.e. yellowing) with age, or some typical effects appeared in most of the patients receiving one of the treatments compared. In very long-term treatments, patients' curiosity becomes very strong after several years and all means of identifications are tried (10). Finally, unblinded final evaluation of cases with code-breaking can be started too early before data corrections or checks are completed.

The attitude to take when faced with this abnormality is not easy: isolated cases can hardly alter the results. They are simply mentioned in the violations section of the report (noting that breaking the code in case of an emergency is an authorized procedure, not a violation).

Systematic cases (including opening code envelopes) will be discussed in detail, trying to analyze whether or not they could influence the outcome and the conclusions.

4.8. Unauthorized co-therapies

If the patient took (with or without a prescription) a therapy which was forbidden by the protocol, three situations should be considered:

• if the unauthorized co-therapy was a safety precaution, the case is evaluated normally and its tolerability results discussed,

• if a redundant co-therapy makes evaluation of efficacy impossible (same indication as the test therapy) and was given at a reasonably effective dose schedule, analyses with and without such cases might be the only reasonable approach,

• if a co-therapy interferes with some efficacy or safety measurements, a separate description and discussion is reserved for their possible influence on results, considering product doses and durations of therapy.

4.9. Multiple admissions

Occasionally a given patient is included twice in the same trial (from the same investigator or even from another one!). This can happen in chronic stable illnesses, or in recurrent episodes, and for diseases observed in succession in two anatomical localizations (two ears, two eyes, etc.). We would recommend in such cases to analyze only the first period in the main efficacy analysis, to give all results in a separate discussion, and to analyze all periods in the safety section.

5. COMPLIANCE

Patient compliance, even when it has been possible to control it, may for some patients be either too little or alternately exagerated. It is very useful to explain poor response in noncompliers, or adverse events in hyper-compliers. Other uses of this information, such as covariance adjustements or exclusion of noncompliers, should only be done cautiously after careful discussion, since this information is obviously available after randomization; compliance might have been influenced by treatment effects. A possible exception is the exclusion of patients, if they are rare, who did not take any dose of the therapy at all, but only if those post-hoc exclusions are balanced between treatment groups in numbers and baseline characteristics. Even in that case a sensitivity analysis (with and without those cases) is advisable.

6. DROP-OUTS AND TREATMENT DISCONTINUATION

A patient can be withdrawn from therapy for various reasons (warranted or not): adverse event, unsatisfactory response, unanticipated health problem leading to a change in treatment priorities, lost or spoiled drug, bad vein for intravenous treatment, or decision by the patient himself...

Even when great care is given to selection of reliable patients, and to motivating them to be followed until the scheduled end of the trial, some patients disappear. If losses are important, the sample attrition not only decreases statistical power but can bias the results. Lost patients can render a group of remainders not random and not comparable.

The different circumstances which lead to cessation of treatment and losses to follow-up and their effects on the analysis of results (6, 8, 9, 11) are described in detail in the chapters "Losses to follow-up, Compliance with therapy and Discontinuation of treatment". Furthemore, the effects on the analysis are also listed in the summary table entitled "Imperfect data".

7. CONCLUSION

A compromise solution must be found for most non evaluable cases. Nevertheless, emphasis should be given to prevention: realistic, detailed and unambiguous protocol and CRFs, selection of rigorous investigators, and compliant patients, training and refresher sessions, frequent monitoring of data, and good organization of appointments, memory reminders. A touch of humanity motivates everyone to participate.

Table I   Imperfect data

General problem	Specific cases	Analyses
Missing values	• There is a previous score	Projection of the preceding score
	• There are redundant data	Estimation based on well-correlated values
	• There is no post-randomization data	Exclusion + discussion
	• Extreme unknown value	See outliers proven to be true
Outlier values	• Recognized to be false	See missing values
	• Proven to be true or • Extreme values outside measurable limits	Non-parametric test if available Otherwise : • "Winsorization" • Estimation based on truncated samples
	• Doubtful values —> independent and "blind" examination	Decide between • "missing values" or • "outlier values proven to be true"

Table I   Imperfect data (cont'd)

General problem	Specific cases	Analyses
Wrongly included (violation of inclusion criteria)	• Diagnosis is clearly erroneous —>independent and "blind" examination	Unarguable error : exclusion + discussion Otherwise: see "doubtful diagnosis"
	• Doubtful diagnosis • Correct diagnosis but criteria for severity (or for stability) not complied with	ITT + subgroup analysis of "perfectly eligible" cases (secondary analysis)
	• Diagnosis not confirmed according to data (or biological samples) : _ collected before randomization	Exclusion + discussion if planned in protocol Otherwise : ITT + subgroup analysis (secondary analysis)
	- collected after randomization - treatment may have affected the results of the diagnostic test	ITT
	- Otherwise ...	ITT + subgroup analysis (secondary analysis)
Cases erroneously not excluded	• Exclusion criteria data not available (e.g. lab test not performed)	ITT
	• Exclusion for "evaluability" - evaluation is available	ITT
	- evaluation is impossible	"See missing data"
	• Exclusion for "risk of loss to follow-up" - patient not lost to follow-up - patient lost to follow-up	ITT See "lost to follow-up"
	• Safety exclusion	ITT
Allocation errors	1) Double-blind trials : • Isolated permutations	By treatment received
	• Mixed-up allocations - blind allocations (inquiry)	"Sensitivity" analysis (by randomization and by treatment received)
	- doubt concerning breaking the blindness	Analysis is jeopardized (tolerability only for each treatment received)
	2) Other cases : • Isolated cases	Analysis by treatment received
	• Systematic (non-blind allocation)	Data usable only for tolerability

Table I Imperfect data (cont'd)

General problem	Specific cases	Analyses
Timing errors	• Small deviations from tolerated ranges	ITT
	• Complete shift in examination program	ITT taking values of results available at closest dates, with discussion
Errors in evaluation		ITT + discussion
Dosing errors	• Objective of trial was to determine optimal dose	ITT + subgroup with correct dose
	• Otherwise	Efficacy: ITT Tolerability: per dose received
Breaking the blindness	• Isolated cases	ITT
	• Systematic (analyse causes)	Discuss possible influence on results
Unauthorized concomitant treatments	• Contraindicated for tolerability reasons	ITT (efficacy), Tolerability analysed separatly
	• Same effect as study medications	Separate analysis (+ discussion on product, dose, duration)
	• May interfere with evaluation criterion	Separate analysis + discussion
Patient entered in trial several times		Main analysis = 1st entry + describe other evaluations
Withdrawal from therapy	• Before minimum duration planned in protocol	"Sensitivity" (with and without)
	Otherwise : - patient not lost to follow-up	ITT
	- patient lost to follow-up	See "lost to follow-up"
Insufficient compliance	• Some subjects did not take any dose of treatment	Exclusion is acceptable + discuss number and influence on comparability
	• Compliance is below a minimum threshold for evaluability (as specified in protocol)	If influence: "sensitivity" (with and without)
	• Other cases	ITT + subsidiary analysis by extent of compliance

Table I Imperfect data (con'd)

General problem	Specific cases	Analyses

Subjects lost to follow-up	• In all cases	Diagram:
		
		- by treatment
		- by timing (figure attached)
		  Description + effect
		  on comparability

	• Life table	Included in analysis until dropout
	• Lost before any evaluation after randomization	Exclusion + discussion
	• Preceding score predictive of final score	Last observation carried forward
	• Preceding trend predictive of final score	Regression from preceding values
	• Some information available on reasons for disappearance	"Success-failure" scores according to causes
	• Other cases	Simulation based on other cases "Sensitivity" + "worst-case scenario"

References

1 Anonymous. Commissariat à l'énergie atomique. Statistiques appliquées à l'exploitation de mesures. Volume 1. Paris: Masson 1978: 93-7.

2 Assenzo JR, Lamborn KR. Documenting the results of a study. In: Buncher CR, Tsay JY. Statistics in the pharmaceutical industry. New York: Marcel Dekker, 1981; 251-300.

3 Bolton S. Pharmaceutical statistics. Ch.10: Transformation and outliers. New York: Marcel Dekker, 1990, 338-361.

4 Carleton RA, Sanders CA, Burack CR. Heparin administration after myocardial infarction. New Engl J Med 1975; 292: 1036-7.

5 Dixon WJ. Processing data for outliers. Biometrics 1953; 9: 74-89.

6 Evans SJW. What can we do with the data we throw away ? Br J Clin Pharmacol 1982; 14: 653-9.

7 Friedewald WT, Schoenberger JA. Overview of recent clinical and methodological advances from clinical trials of cardiovascular diseases. Controlled Clinical Trials 1982; 3: 259-270.

8 Friedman LM, Furberg CD, DeMets DL. Fundamentals of clinical trials. Littleton: PSG Publishing Company, 1985.

9 Gould AL. A new approach to the analysis of clinical drug trials with withdrawals. Biometrics 1980; 36: 721-7.

10 Howard J. Whittemore J, Hoover J. Panos M. How blind was the patient blind in the AMIS ? Clin Pharmacol Ther 1982; 32: 543-53.

11 Leber P. Form and content of NDA reviews: strategies for the efficacy analysis. Food and Drug Administration (Memorandum), Nov 5, 1985.

12 May GS, DeMets DL, Friedman LM, Furberg C, Passamani E. The randomized clinical trial: bias in analysis. Circulation 1981; 64: 669-73.

13 Peto R, Pike MC, Armitage NE et al. Designs and anlysis of randomized clinical trials requiring prolonged observation of each patient. I. Introduction and design. Br J Cancer 1976; 34: 585-618.

14 Pocock SJ. Clinical trials: a practical approach. Chichester: John Wiley and Sons, 1983, 176-87.

15 Wolf GT, Makuch RW. Editorial: a classification system for protocol deviations in clinical trials. Cancer Clin Trials 1980; 3: 101-3.

15 - Confirmatory analysis
of the principal evaluation criterion

SUMMARY

Once all the data from a clinical trial have been collected, before comparing the results of treatments, it is essential to describe the data and to check for treatment group comparability.

The statistical methods used to analyze the results will depend on a number of factors including:

• the nature of the variables:
- binary or dichotomous variables (e.g. success or failure) can be analyzed by several methods allowing comparison of frequencies;
- ordered classification or ranked variables (e.g. good, fair, poor);
- normally distributed or Gaussian distributed variables for which there are several parametric tests;
- quantitative non-normally distributed variables can be analyzed using non-parametric tests;

• the number of treatments compared;

• the experimental design;

• additional factors taken into account for the analysis (e.g. initial degree of severity).

In this chapter, in tables and comments, we list the tests that can be applied to commonly encountered situations and explain how they should be used.

The life-table method is used in clinical trials where patients are included at different times, followed up for variable periods of time and where the evaluation criterion is the time it takes to reach an "endpoint" or critical event such as death, a complication or recurrence of disease.

Multivariate methods are used to take into account several variables simultaneously. These methods can resolve the problem of redundant variables, i.e. those which are correlated to a greater or lesser degree. However, a priori, multivariate methods attribute the same importance to all the variables, regardless of their true clinical importance and paradoxically, they are some-times less powerful than tests performed on the same variables considered individually.

A statistical interaction (difference depending on centers, periods or other factors) sometimes leads to restrictions in the interpretation of results. Equivalence between the two treatments can only be affirmed if the confi-dence interval is within narrow limits.

Meta-analysis allows results of several trials to be combined retrospectively if their data are compatible and of sufficient quality.

All the data from a clinical trial should be checked as soon as possible after it has been made available in order to detect any errors, omissions or "unli-kely" results. It is only after this important work has been done that the data are submitted to statistical analysis which consists of three major phases: *description* of the data, the study of group *comparability* and the *comparison* of the treatments for efficacy and safety. Prior to this, decisions concerning imperfect data must have been made and justified (see preceding chapter). All these steps will be presented in a trial report for which it is advisable to follow a standard model (105). The statistical methods used should be chosen carefully. There are many methods from which to choose. One should avoid indiscerningly using just any simple, wellknown method if other methods, more appropriate for the experimental design used or the type of data collected are available. It is equally disastrous to perform a perfunctory statistical analysis on difficult to acquire data using all-purpose methods, as it is to conceal worthless data behind an esoteric and pompous facade of seemingly impressive calculations.

It is not our intent to describe all the available statistical methods but simply to provide the reader with some guidelines which will help him to choose the methods most appropriate for his particular problem.

In the discussion that follows, we assume that the reader is familiar with the concepts of probability, type 1 and type 2 errors, the null and alternative hypotheses, statistical significance, one-tailed and two-tailed tests and experimental design. All these terms have been explained in detail in pre-vious chapters.

1. DESCRIPTION OF DATA

All the data collected must first be presented clearly in the form of lists, tables, histograms or graphs. For each subject, the changes in the study parameters with time should be examined. For each quantitative variable, maximum and minimum values should be investigated. This sometimes leads to the discovery of errors (outlier values) previously unnoticed.

The means and variances (or their non-parametric equivalents, medians and quantiles) will be calculated together with the confidence intervals.

This preliminary step of the analysis may appear simplistic and tedious, but it is in fact fundamental and very instructive in regard to errors that should be avoided and the interpretation of the results.

2. DIFFERENCES BETWEEN GROUPS

Even when the groups have been correctly randomized, allocation of the treatments by chance may produce an imbalance for one or several factors that have some influence on the result - age, initial status or concomitant disorders - for example. One possible way of compensating for this imbalance is to "post-stratify" the groups but this may make the analysis and interpretation of the results difficult.

It is therefore important to check whether the groups designated by random allocation are reasonably similar (36). Of course, one can compare the groups for any number of characteristics but the greater the number of tests performed, the more likely it is that one of them will turn out "significant".

From a practical standpoint, a problem arises when differences are found that may markedly affect the criterion of evaluation. It is more serious still to remain unaware of such differences. It is simply common sense to restrict the comparisons to variables which are likely to bear a relationship to the result and to disregard the others. If sufficient thought has gone into the planning of the protocol, only "relevant" data will have beeen collected in any case. In addition, if certain patients who were lost to follow-up are excluded from some of the analyses, comparability should be checked with and without the *incomplete* cases. Lastly, one should be wary about interpreting comparability tests in small groups of subjects as such tests may not be "statistically significant" even when there are striking differences between the groups.

Initial dissimilarity between the groups will be interpreted differently depending on whether it is favorable or unfavorable to the treatment which turns out to be the best.

When studying group comparability, although there may be no differences between simple variables, it may nevertheless be important in some cases to ensure that there is no imbalance between *combinations* of these variables. For example, a trial comparing two treatments may include two groups that are comparable for age and sex, considered individually, but one of the groups may contain more old men and young women than the other group.

3. COMPARISON OF RESULTS ON EFFICACY

3.1. Factors in the choice of statistical methods

The choice of an appropriate statistical method depends on several factors including:

- the experimental design and the number of treatments compared (and also possibly the number of planned treatment comparisons 2 by 2 when there are 3 or more treatments. This should not be done by separate tests but by "contrasts" breaking-down the global analysis (36, 41, 76, 79, 117).

- the nature of the variables: binary, dichotomous or non-continuous variables ("yes" or "no" response), semi-quantitative variables continuous (ideally forming a "normal" or *Gaussian distribution*) with equal or unequal variances;

- the number of subjects: exact tests for small samples, asymptotic tests for large samples;

- concomitant variables or "covariates" that we wish to take into account;

- the number of evaluations: before and after treatment, repeated measurements during treatment.

However, the choice of the statistical methods which depend on the results are criticizable if they have not been decided before the start of the trial, and at least before decoding of randomization, particularly:
• selected "analyzable" cases,
• choosing a method that combines variables,
• introducing "post-stratifications" or using "covariates",
• analyzing subgroups separately.

All situations have been listed in a table with references. In this table we have also indicated the main conditions for the validity of the test under consideration. The references quoted are not intended to indicate the original description of a method or its demonstration, but rather to direct the reader to descriptions that can be used in practice, and as often a possible in standard manuals.

3.2. Binary or dichotomous variables

When the criterion for assessing a result is expressed as a "yes" or "no" answer (e.g. success or failure, death or survival, recurrence or no recurrence, complication or no complication, presence or absence of side-effects, etc.) the result may be recorded in terms of the frequency, proportion or percentage of favorable or unfavorable outcomes.

It must be pointed out that this type of analysis cannot be applied to questions where doubt is possible (i.e. questions that may be answered by "yes" "no" or "maybe", nor to questions that call for graded answers ("none, some, many" or "never, sometimes, always").

The "yes" or "no" answer is the least elaborate form of response and it would be disastrous to reduce a quantitative or semi-quantitative variable to this simple form as the statistical comparison would be considerably weakened by *loss of information*.

Table I illustrates the main tests that can be used for analyzing a dichotomous response in a parallel group or crossover trial. This table also includes methods that permit analysis of dichotomous results while taking another factor of classification into account.

Table I   Dichotomous variables

Situations		Tests	References	Remarks
Parallel groups	**2 treatments A and B** Contingency table (2X2) A B Success Failure	$\chi 2$ with correction for continuity*	(36)	Use of this test is questionable if discontinuity is substantial (expected number small in at least one of the 4 cells of the table)(19)
		Exact probability Two-tailed test	(35, 36) (1)	Calculation difficult if there are large numbers of subjects
		log-likelihood test with correction for continuity	(103, 118)	Less limited by disconti- nuity than the $\chi 2$ test
	≥ **3 treatments** Contingency table (2 x k)	$\chi 2$	(36)	Partitioning of the table (to compare one treatment to several others, or two treatments or two groups of treatments between themselves) is possible if the tables thus obtained are orthogonal (41)
	Treatments 1 2 ... k Success Failure	log-likelihood test	(103, 118)	
		Exact probability Hybrid method: exact + asymptotic probability (coexistence of small and large number of patients)	(38, 75, 81) (3)	
	Repeated response several times in the same subject		(65)	

* Yates's correction, or better still corrections of Kendall-Stuart or of Cochran : the mean of the calculated value for $\chi 2$ and of the nearest lower that can be obtained with the same marginal totals (total number per treatment and total number per result) (21, 46).

Table I   Dichotomous variables (cont'd)

Situations		Tests	References	Remarks
Within patient trial	**2 treatments**	Binomial test	(36)	Recommended for small samples
		McNemar's test	(36)	Large samples
		Gart's method	(40)	Allowing taking into consideration an order effect (different efficacy if treatment is administered first or second)
	≥ 3 treatments	Cochran's Q test	(19)	Applicable only if sample is not too small (28)
Analysis taking into account a factor other than treatment and result, and in particular a "prognostic" factor for stratification	**2 treatments**	Combination of several 2x2 tables	(69)	Several methods depending on the hypothesis being tested
	≥3 treatments	Combination of several tables n x m: Mantel-Haenzel's test	(71)	
		3-dimensional contingency table* - χ^2 analysis - partitioning	(59, 117) (34, 73) (103)	Makes it possible to test 2 by 2 the 3 dimensions in the table of contingencies and one term of interaction.
Dose-effect relationship			(42)	
Several classifications	**General methods for analyzing different situations**	Linear models, or log linear "logistic models"	(23, 45)	

* For example :
• treatments A, B, C
• within each group there are two subgroups ("mild" and "severe" forms of the disease),
• for each treatment either : sucess or failure.

3.3. Classifying results into several ordinal categories

When a result has been characterized by grades (for example very good, good, fair or nil), the tests used to analyze the data should take into account the ordinal nature of the classes. These tests are listed in table II.

Theoretically, a distinction should be made between a purely qualitative classification, where the results are distributed into several classes in no particular order and a classification in which the results are graded (for example more or less favorable outcome of a treatment). In practice, when one analyzes the results of a therapeutic trial, the first situation never arises.

A particular case involves the occurrence of recurrent events for which the number of episodes is the assessment criterion (111).

Table II
Ordered classification
(ordered responses)

Situations	Tests	References	Remarks
Ordered treatments (increasing doses) 2 parallel groups	• «Yates's method»	(119)	Quantitative classification
	• Bartholomew's method	(4, 36)	Ordinal classification but quantification impossible
Other cases	Generalised linear model	(23, 26, 45, 80)	Allows a wide variety of tests, requires matrix algebra and a powerful computer
Semi-quantitative scores 2 parallel groups	Krauth's method	(67, 108)	
Cross-over trial	Preference scale (-3 à +3)	(92)	
Scores transformed depending on their frequency in a reference population (e.g. placebo group)	RIDIT transformation	(36)	
Analysis of changes in discontinuous scores (before-after treatment)	• «Generalized Kappa»	(62)	Comparison of square tables (one per treatment)
	• Stratification according to initial score	(32)	

3.4. Normally distributed (or Gaussian distributed variables), parametric tests.

When the variable to be analyzed is quantifiable (measurement of a continuous phenomenon), if we can postulate that the variable follows a *Gaussian or normal distribution*[*], we can use parametric tests based on this feature. Parametric tests have the advantage of being more "powerful" i.e. more sensitive to differences in mean values for a given number of cases. There are also several types of parametric tests which can handle complex experimental designs or concomitant variables and their "interactions" (variable differences in different subgroups).

It is therefore tempting to assume a normal distribution for the variables to be analyzed.

3.4.1. Problems raised by the hypothesis of "normality"

• Robustness of the tests

In theory, a parametric test gives a false result if it is applied to a non-Gaussian distribution. The "less normal" the distribution, the greater the error.

It is impossible to determine the degree of non-normality which produces an acceptable margin of error in the final calculation of probability.

However, all the parametric tests are not equally sensitive to non-normality. The t test applied to two groups of equal sample sizes is far less sensitive than the other methods (9, 82).

• Type of distribution

There are several types of non-normal distributions. One is asymmetry, that is to say more values far above the mean than far below the mean or vice versa. Another type of non-normal distribution is non-normal *kurtosis* which refers to "peaked" or flat distribution.

In practice, from the viewpoint of parametric tests, the most unfavorable types of non-normal distribution appear to be bimodality and extreme asymmetry (9).

• Transforming variables

When dealing with an overtly *non-normal* distribution, it is sometimes possible to transform the variables (by taking their logarithms for example), so as to arrive at an approximate normal distribution. However, since it is possible to make an unlimited number of transformations, the choice must not be made in light of the treatment results, but only as a function of the correction of the distribution obtained.

• The influence of sample size

Another particular factor allows the use of parametric tests when these assumptions are violated, namely that the inaccuracy of these tests diminishes as sample size increases.

It is possible, therefore, to adopt parametric tests for large samples, for example, "more than 30" cases, as is sometimes recommended. However,

[*] The precise definition of this term (which is based on a mathematical function) implies among other things that the distribution is symmetrical and that extreme values at each tail of the distribution are fewer and fewer in number.

it is not possible to define a fixed number of cases beyond which the distribution can be disregarded since *the sample size for which non-normality can be ignored* depends on the degree of non-normality. In one example of bimodal distribution studied by Bradley (9), a reasonable level of approximation (arbitrarily set at $\pm 20\%$ for the probability calculation of the test around the limit of significance $\alpha = 0.05$) was reached only when the sample size exceeded 1000 !

• Influence of the significance level

The "robustness" of a test also decreases as the significance level becomes lower and lower. In the above example, for $\alpha = 0.01$, the 20% approximation for p would have required 4000 cases.

Table III
Gaussian variables

Situations		Tests	References	Remarks
Parallel groups	**2 treatments**	Equal variances: t test Unequal variances: Welch's test	(117) (113)	The equality of 2 variances can be tested by their ratio (use the higher value as a denominator and take as the lower limit of significance the value "F" corresponding to $\frac{\alpha}{2}$ for a significance level α).
	≥ 3 treatments	Equal variances: analysis of variance Unequal variances: analysis of variance with heterogeneous variances multiple comparisons	(117) (12)	Equality of several variances can be tested by several methods, Levenne's method in particular (13)
Within-patient trial	**2 treatments**	Analysis of variance: -period factor -treatment factor -interaction period x treatment	(10, 44, 51, 112)	
	≥ 3 treatments	ANOVA for: -latin square -incomplete blocks	(117)	See chapter on "experimental design"
Trial with stratification		Multiple-way ANOVA (numerous models adapted to different situations)	(30, 94, 117)	
Repeated measurements		ANOVA for repeated measurements Multivariate analysis	(43, 63) (47)	
Dose-effect relationship		Test of ordered means Test for the smallest dose different from control	(73, 78) (115, 116)	
Analysis taking into account a quantitative variable independent of treatment (e.g. pretreatment value)		Analysis of covariance	(54, 117)	

• Usefulness of a test of normality

It is possible to use statistical tests for *normality*. These tests enable us to reject the hypothesis that a given set of variables is normally distributed. The various methods available for testing the normality of the distribution are not equally sensitive to different types of *non-normality* (88, 100).

These tests are relatively insensitive when the number of subjects is small. If, on the other hand, such tests are applied to large samples, the hypothesis of normality will nearly always be rejected since the true Gaussian distribution is an abstract entity from which "natural" distributions always depart to a greater or lesser degree. *We thus find ourselves faced with the following paradox: the probability of rejecting the hypothesis of normality increases as the number of subjects becomes larger, i.e. when non-normality becomes less of a problem.*

3.4.2. "Parametric" tests applicable to Gaussian variables

The main methods used in therapeutic trials are outlined in *table III*.

For analysis of variance (abbreviated ANOVA), there are a number of available methods, and only those that correspond to the most frequently encountered situations can be mentioned here.

• The prerequisites for analysis of variance include the following:

- random allocation of treatments;
- Gaussian distribution;
- equal variances (although there are models that take into account unequal variances (12);
- additivity of the factors (which can be tested, if for each combination of factors, more than one case is available) (103).

Transformation of variables (logarithmic in particular) often allowing correction of violations of assumptions

• The case of multiple comparisons in an analysis of variance

When one of the classifications analyzed by ANOVA consists of more than two classes, it may be useful to perform *multiple comparisons* to single out the sources of significant differences. These simultaneous comparisons or "contrasts" (e.g. of treatments taken pairwise) cannot be made by independent tests and they require special techniques. There are a number of techniques available, each adapted to a different situation (76, 79). Some of the most commonly used include:
- multiple comparisons versus a single control group or Dunnett's tests (28, 29, 30, 31);
- predetermined pairwise comparisons or Bonferroni's method (76, 102);
- comparisons decided *a posteriori*: method of Scheffé (93), Duncan (27, 48), Newman-Keuls (117), etc.

Figure 1a
"After" treatment values not correlated with "before" treatment values → tests on "after" values

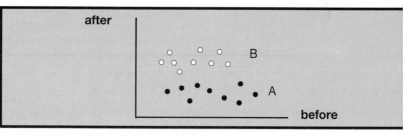

Figure 1b
The "before-after" treatment relationship is a straight line with a slope = 1→ test on the differences.

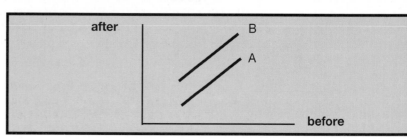

Figure 1c
The differences between treatments are proportional to the pretreatment values → test on percentage variation.

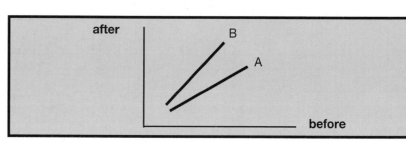

Figure 1d
Before/after relationship is the same for both treatments (slope ≠ 1) → analysis of covariance

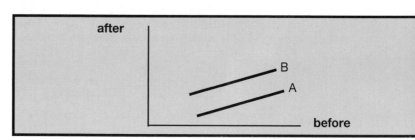

• "Before and after" measurements

In the very common situation where a measurement before and after treatment is available, the analysis can be done in several different ways (57):
- either disregard the pretreatment measurement and analyze *only the posttreatment data*. In doing this we are implicitly formulating the hypothesis that the measurement after treatment is uncorrelated (in practice, coefficient of correlation $r < 0.5$) with the pretreatment value (figure 1a);
- or, another approach is to compare the differences ("before" and "after")

We are thus assuming that the regressions between the measurements before and after treatment are straight lines with a slope of 1 (figure 1b), or that the "before-after" difference is not proportional to the pretreatment value (68);

- lastly, we can also analyze the percentage of variation (or equivalently, the *ratio* "value after treatment/value before treatment"). The assumption with this method is that the differences are proportional to the pretreatment values (figure 1c), that is to say that the percentage of variation is the same, regardless of the initial score. This may be termed differently by saying that we are assuming that a large variation over a high initial score has the same significance as a small variation over a low initial score[*].

- analysis of covariance may also be used (the initial value of the criterion is considered as a "covariate").

This method assumes that the regression of the values *after treatment* base on values *before treatment* are identical (in particular, if the regression is a linear one, that the lines will have the same slope) (figure 1d).

• Influence of other variables

Analysis of covariance can also be used to consider one or several initial variables (possibly in addition to the pretreatment value of the evaluation criterion on which the analysis is based).

It renders comparisons more sensitive by subtracting from the variance of the evaluation criterion the contribution due to covariates. The use of a covariate increases the sensitivity of the comparison only if it influences the outcome (37), otherwise it reduces the sensitivity. The choice of covariates can influence the result (2, 5, 6, 14, 18, 33, 74, 83, 99). Thus it is more acceptable if it is made a priori rather than a posteriori, and because of a correlation, with the evaluation criterion rather than to correct an initial dissimilarity.

• Linear models

Lastly, a generalized linear model can be used to handle all cases of variance and covariance analysis in the same system (20, 80).

3.5. Continuous non-normal variables, non-parametric tests

When we are not sure if a test designed for normal variables is applicable to a given set of data, we can use "non-parametric" tests, which have fewer assumptions.

Non-parametric tests are, however, slightly less powerful. Their *relative power* (ratio of the number of cases required to demonstrate a given difference with two tests) with two-sample "rank" tests, for example, is 3/Π or approximately 0.95) which is very acceptable (77). The "loss" of efficacy is certainly less crucial than the error resulting from violations of hypotheses with the use of "parametric" tests.

[*] In this case we often perform the analysis on the *logarithm* of the before/after ratio so that the variances are not proportional to the means. Then, the means shown in tables and graphs should preferably be the *geometric* means : n[th] root of the product of n variables, or the antilogarithm of the mean of the logarithms (96).

Unfortunately, non-parametric tests offer far more limited possibilities with regard to complex experimental designs, repeated measurements, missing data and concomitant variables. The main non-parametric methods are shown in table IV.

Table IV
Non-parametric tests

Situations		Tests	References	Remarks
Parallel groups	**2 treatments**	Mann and Whitney's test Kolmogorov-Smirnov's test Terry-Hoeffdings test Fisher's randomization test *	(9, 101) (9, 101) (67, 110) (101)	
	≥3 treatments	Kruskall-Wallis's test Pitman's randomization test	(9, 101) (86)	Pairwise comparison: Steel's method (76, 117)
Within-patient trial	**2 treatments**	Test taking into account: -period effect -treatment effect -period-treatment interaction	(64)	
	≥3 treatments	Friedman's test Pitman's test (*) for paired data	(9, 101)	Contrast: Anderson's method (79)
Factorial design			(70, 95)	Includes tests for interaction and contrasts
Repeated measurements		Different models of ANOVA	(60, 61, 63, 90)	If variances are unequal over time: corrections (43, 61) or comparisons of "smooth-ened out" curves (90)
Dose-effect relationship			(52, 53, 98)	
Analysis taking into account a covariate		Non-parametric analysis of covariance	(89)	

* "Randomization" or "permutation" tests (Fisher, Pitman) are more powerful than rank (ordinal) tests but entail considerable calculation difficulties when there are a large number of data. They are of particular interest when there are many ties.

3.6. Life-table methods (49)

When the evaluation criterion for the effects of the treatments compared is the time it takes to reach an "end-point" (dichotomous variable such as death, relapse, cure, discontinuation of treatment or development of an adverse event, etc.) *which may or may not occur during the observation period*, we can calculate a survival curve to compare the rates of and times to this end-point between the different groups.

This method is based on the following principles:

• the observation time for all the subjects is not necessarily the same. Participants may enter the trial successively at any point. The trial may end on a fixed date. Thus, the first patients will have been followed up for longer than later entries into the study;

• the survival rate is calculated for different follow-up periods:
- either for given periods of time - months or years - *from the date when the patients entered the trial*: actuarial method (7, 25);
- or at the time when each endpoint occurs (58);

The "survival" rate is evaluated stepwise for successive time-points ("survival" as used here does not necessarily mean non-death but rather the non-occurrence of the particular event defining the end-point). At each time-point, subjects who have been in the study long enough to reach that time-point are taken into account (in other words, *fewer and fewer subjects are evaluated at each step*);

• subjects who are lost to follow-up for a *known reason* (bearing no relation to the end-point) are included in the analysis for the time during which they were observed). If the life-table is calculated for *time intervals*, they are arbitrarily counted as having been observed for half of the interval during which they were lost to follow-up;

• for subjects lost to follow-up for an *unknown reason*, we may either formulate a pessimistic hypothesis (they are all considered as having reached the endpoint, for example death), an optimistic hypothesis (they are considered as not having reached the endpoint), or a neutral hypothesis (they are considered as having reached the endpoint with the same frequency as the other subjects). In the latter case, participants are omitted from the calculation form the time when they were lost to follow-up;

• the calculation may include some initial variables - *or covariates* - with prognostic value (such as age or severity of the illness, for example). This allows for the fact that the subjects do not *a priori* have the same chance of reaching the endpoint, independently of the treatments they receive (17, 24);

• the life-tables for several treatments may be compared by using the appropriate tests, which depend on whether the tables are drawn up for given periods (72) of time or according to the actual dates of reaching the endpoints (84). Sequential methods of analysis also can be used (114);

• lastly, it may be useful to detect a difference that varies in time; for example, a higher mortality rate for one treatment early in the observation period, and a lower mortality rate later (107).

3.7. Multidimensional or multivariate methods

When several variables have to be included *simultaneously* in a calculation, correlations between these variables must be taken into account. Two strongly related variables are to some extent "duplicative" (they are redundant). Some variables provide very little extra information.

Multivariate statistical methods (22, 87, 109) must therefore consider the *covariances* of each variable in relation to every other variable. The most commonly used methods for comparing the effects of two or more treatments are multivariate tests with normal or Gaussian variables. For comparing two parallel groups, Hotelling's T2 test is appropriate, while for other more complex investigations, multivariate analysis of variance (MANOVA) or of covariance can be used.

• Multivariate methods formulate hypotheses about the variables which are sometimes difficult to verify, in particular, the multivariate normal distribution, and the equality of the variances and covariances.

• The multivariate analyses do not solve every problem and can even create their own specific difficulties.

- *A priori*, multivariate methods attribute the same importance to all the variables. In the analysis itself, however, the variables are, of course, given different weights, but only on statistical criteria (resulting from correlation with the other variables) and not on their relative clinical importance (34).

- Multivariate methods are often less powerful than tests performed on the individual variables; the latter may show a significant difference in cases where the global multivariate test does not.

This so-called "*Rao's* paradox" can be attributed to the fact that multivariate tests may be *less robust* with regard to the underlying assumptions such as normality of distribution or equality of the variances (66).

• In addition to the methods used to compare two or more groups, other multivariate methods are sometimes used in clinical trials:

- Principal component analysis makes possible to compose other variables from non-independent multiple variables, which are *linear combinations* of the former (i.e. the sum of the variables, each multiplied by a different weighting coefficient) and are not correlated with each other.

The *combinations obtained* in this manner are then ranked in order of variance of the initial variables they represent.

The first components therefore *provide much more information* than the last ones, which can then be ignored. This enables us to simplify the data. This method is sometimes used - particularly for rating scales - in the following way: the "weights" are calculated from an analysis of the data collected from the subjects *before they receive their treatment*. The weights are then applied to the variables *after treatment* to demonstrate differences due to the treatments.

- *Methods of factorial analysis* of which principal components analysis is a particular case makes it possible to use the initial variables to compose independent factors for which pre-specified weights are taken into account. These methods therefore permit representing the data *both* in simplified form and with pre-specified weights. They are sometimes completed by transformation of the factors ("Varimax rotation") so that fewer variables are more strongly represented in each factor, which makes the interpretation of their clinical significance easier. The coefficients of a previous factorial analysis (carried out with data from a previous study) are sometimes used to calculate these same factors on the data of a clinical trial, and to serve as an evaluation criterion.

- Discriminant analysis methods use distinct groups to calculate the best linear combination of the variables (collected from the subjects of these groups), which maximizes the difference or "distance" between these groups. Discriminant analysis methods are sometimes used in an attempt to distinguish "responders" from "non responders" (unfavorable results) on the basis of data from a clinical trial. If the distinction proves satisfactory, we can hope to "predict" the results of the treatment, guiding other investigators or physicians in better treatment selections for study participants or individual patients.

- *Multiple regression methods* make it possible to predict a quantitative variable from a set of *"predictive"* variables. They are also used to attempt to predict responses to treatments, when these responses can be expressed numerically as an improvement "score".

If the predicted variable is a *probability* (for example, the chance of surviving or not), then we use a *logistical* multiple regression based on exponential transformation), the "response" being beween zero and one.

3.8. Interactions

It is sometimes desirable to investigate not only the influence of concomitant variables on the variability of results but also their influence on the *differences between treatments being compared. Here we are dealing with interactions*, the statistical significance of which can be tested. At the limit, the differences between treatments may be in opposite directions if analysis is based on the values of a concomitant variable (*qualitative or "cross-over" interaction*). Important examples of interaction can be quoted: "center-treatment" interaction in a multicenter trial (variable differences between treatments in different centers), "time-treatment" interaction (variable differences between treatments at different times), "subgroups-treatment" interaction (variable differences between treatments for different subgroups). Interpretation of this last case should be cautious and in particular it should take into account *the number of subdivisions tried or possible*, and not only those that appear to reveal an interesting difference. It is incorrect, in a confirmatory approach, to attempt to single out "significant" combinations if an overall interaction test is "non-significant" (85).

Generally speaking, interpretation of an interaction should take several factors into account:

- the direction of the differences of differences,
- their magnitude,
- their biological plausibility if a cause is found or suspected,
- the number of interactions tested.

A significant and clinically important interaction can lead to a restriction in the generalization of results.

4. EQUIVALENCE

Often in the comparison of two active drugs (generally, a new drug and a standard drug) the objective is not to demonstrate that one is better than the other, but rather to prove that the new drug is just about as effective as the existing treatment.

The analysis begins by a test of efficacy, always a two-sided test, which most often is not significant. This result alone does not make it possible to conclude in the equivalence of the two drugs. In addition, it must be demonstrated that any difference is not large, i.e. is less than the maximum difference Δ. To show that the two are equivalent, this limit must have been defined a priori in the study protocol.

Δ is an arbitrary value which must be convincing and therefore the smallest possible value. A compromise is necessary between Δ which is too high (equivalence not convincing) or too low (requiring a utopian number of cases). On the basis of this compromise, the widest possible consensus is necessary (clinical credibility, economic feasibility, acceptability by the drug registration authorities).

The most widely used method to exclude a difference greater than Δ is the calculation of the *confidence interval of the difference* (39, 104): the extent of values compatible with data on one side and the other of the observed difference. The range of this interval is proportional to the variability of results and is inversely proportional to the number of cases.

If this interval lies entirely between $+\Delta$ and $-\Delta$ equivalence of the two treatments can be accepted within the extent of Δ. If not, a doubt persists concerning their equivalence (see chapter 2 figure 3b). If it overlaps only one of the two limits ($+\Delta$ or $-\Delta$), it enables exclusion of a major difference in the opposite direction to the one observed. In some cases, a test of rejection of the alternative hypothesis can be used (40, 50, 97).

5. META-ANALYSIS

Meta-analysis can be of use in verifying retrospectively whether the combination of several trials, whose results are not significant, make it possible to obtain overall significance, or to know if significance obtained in an isolated trial should be attenuated by other trials for which the difference does not seem to be significant (41).

This method consists of several steps (8, 16, 55, 56, 91).

5.1. Objective

Definition of the objective of the meta-analysis most often is the same as the principal hypothesis of individual trials. Sometimes it is an explanatory type of analysis intended to generate other hypotheses.

5.2. Compilation

Compilation of all trials with the same objective (the same treatments and a protocol that is compatible) must be done. This is easy for trials that have been published but necessitates searching for unpublished results whose conclusions are often unfavorable. Searching for abstracts from congresses is very useful to make the most possible comprehensive determination of all publicized research. But the knowledge of specialists concerned with the disorder under study is a supplementary approach if a systematic registry is not available.

5.3. Quality assessment

Quality can be assessed by using a list of items and an overall score which generally is based on weighting of items (15, 106). This score enables screening for the exclusion of trials or for making a separate analysis.

One should not forget the arbitrary nature of the weighting process and therefore of this screening.

5.4. A single analysis combining the chosen trials

Depending on the information available, the statistical analysis combines:
- either individual data (the ideal situation but one difficult to obtain) (71)
- or the results of tests in each trial;
- or the test probability only (11, 35).

5.5. Interpretation

The principal statistical test and the confidence interval of the difference make it possible to conclude in the existence of a difference, and of its size. If there is trial-treatment interaction, the results cannot be considered as homogeneous and therefore the generalization is limited unless a plausible explanation is found. As always, any other observation on accessory points requires independent confirmation.

References

1   Armitage P. Statistical methods in medical research. Oxford: Blackwell Scientific Publications, 1971.

2   Armitage P. Importance of prognostic factors in the analysis of data from clinical trials. Controlled Clinical Trials 1981; *1*: 347-53.

3   Baglivo J, Olivier D, Pagano M. Methods for the analysis of contingency tables with large and small cell counts. J Amer Stat Assoc 1988; *83*: 1006-13.

4   Bartholomew DJ. A test of homogeneity for ordered alternatives. I Biometrika 1959; *46*: 36-48. II Biometrika 1959; *46*: 328-35.

5   Beach ML, Meier P. Choosing covariates in the analysis of clinical trials. Controlled Clinical Trials 1989; *10*: 161S-75S.

6   Begg CB. Suspended judgment. Significance tests of covariate imbalance in clinical trials. Controlled Clinical Trials 1990; *11*: 223-25.

7   Berkson J, Gage RP. Calculation of survival rates for cancer. Proc Staff Meet Mayo Clinic 1950; *25*: 270-86.

8   Boissel JP, Blanchard J, Panak E et al. Considerations for the meta-analysis of randomized clinical trials. Controlled Clinical Trials 1989; *10*: 254-81.

9   Bradley JV. Distribution-free statistical tests. Englewood Cliffs NJ: Prentice-Hall Inc, 1968.

10 Brown BW Jr. The cross-over experiment for clinical trials. Biometrics 1980; *36*: 69-79.

11 Brown MB. A method of combining non-independent one-sided tests of significance. Biometrics 1975; *31*: 987-92.

12 Brown MB, Forsythe AB. The ANOVA and multiple comparisons for data with heterogeneous variances. Biometrics 1974; *30*: 719-24.

13 Brown MB, Forsythe AB. Robust tests for the equality of variances. J Amer Statist Assoc 1974; *69*: 364-7.

14 Canner PL. Covariate adjustment of treatment effects in clinical trials. Controlled Clinical Trials 1991; *12*: 359-66.

15 Chalmers TC, Smith H, Blackburn B et al. A method for assessing the quality of a randomized control trial. Controlled Clinical Trials 1981; *2*: 3-49.

16 Chalmers TC. Problems induced by meta-analyses. Statistics in Medicine 1991; *10*: 971-80.

17 Chastang C, Byar D, Piantadosi S. A quantitative study of the bias in estimating the treatment effect caused by omitting a balanced covariate in survival models. Statistics in Medicine 1988; *7*: 1243-55.

18 Crager MR. Analysis of covariance in parallel group clinical trials with pre-treatment baselines. Biometrics 1987; *43*: 895-901.

19 Cochran WG. Some methods of strengthening the common χ^2 tests. Biometrics 1954; *10*: 451-71.

20 Cohen J. Multiple regression as a general data-analytic system. Psychol Bulletin 1968; *70*: 426-43.

21 Conover WJ. Some reasons for not using the Yates continuity correction on 2 x 2 contingency tables. J Amer Statist Assoc 1974; *69*: 374-81.

22 Cooley WW, Lohnes PR. Multivariate data analysis. New York: John Wiley and Sons, 1971.

23 Cox DR. The analysis of binary data. London: Chapman and Hall, 1970.

24 Cox DR. Regression models and life-tables. J R Statist Soc 1972; *34*: 187-202.

25 Cutler SJ, Ederer FE. Maximum utilization of the life-table method in analyzing survival. J Chronic Diseases 1958; *8*: 699-712.

26 Downing RW. The application of log linear models to the analysis of cross-classification data generated by single and multiple drug trials. In: Levine J, ed. Coordinating clinical trials in psychopharmacology. Rockville: NIMH 1979: 101-39.

27 Duncan DB. Multiple range and multiple F tests. Biometrics 1955; *11*: 1-42.

28 Dunnett CW. A multiple comparison for comparing several treatments with a control. J Amer Statist Assoc 1955; *50*: 1096-121.

29 Dunnett CW. New tables for multiple comparison with a control. Biometrics 1964; *20*: 482-91.

30 Dunnett CW. Pairwise multiple comparisons in the homogeneous variance, unequal sample size case. J Amer Statist Assoc 1980; *75*: 789-95.

31 Dunnett CW, Tamhane AC. Step-down multiple tests for comparing treatments with a control in unbalanced one-way layouts. Statistics in Medicine 1991; *10*: 939-47.

32 Elton RA, Tiplady B. Mild, moderate, severe. The statistical analysis of short ordinal scales. Neuropharmacology 1980; *19*: 1239.

33 Enas GG, Enas NE, Spradlin CT et al. Baseline comparability in clinical trials: prevention of "post study anxiety". Drug Information Journal 1990; *24*: 541-8.

34 Feinstein AR. Clinical biostatistics XXI. A primer of concepts, phrases, and procedures in the statistical analysis of multiple variables. Clin Pharmacol Ther 1973; *14*: 462-77.

35 Fischer RA. Statistical methods for research workers. 14th edition. Edinburgh: Oliver and Boyd, 1970: 99-101.

36 Fleiss JL. Statistical methods for rates and proportions. New York: John Wiley and Sons, 1973.

37 Forsythe AB. Post hoc decision to use a covariate. J Chron Dis 1977; *30*: 61-4.

38 Freeman GH, Halton JH. Note on an exact treatment of contingency, goodness of fit and other problems of significance. Biometrika 1951; *38*: 141-9.

39 Gardner MJ, Altamn DG. Statistics with confidence. Confidence intervals and statistical guidelines. London: British Medical Journal (Publisher), 1989.

40 Gart JJ. An exact test for comparing matched proportion in cross-over designs. Biometrika 1969; *56*: 75-80.

41 Goldman L, Feinstein AR. Anticoagulants and myocardial infarction. The problem of pooling, drowning, and floating. Ann Int Med 1979; *90*: 92-4.

42 Graubard BI, Korn EL. Choice of column scores for testing independence in ordered 2 x k contingency tables. Biometrics 1987; *43*: 471-6.

43 Greenhouse SW, Geisser S. On methods in the analysis of profile data. Psychometrika 1959; *24*: 95-112.

44 Grizle JE. The two-period change-over design and its use in clinical trials. Biometrics 1965; *21*: 467-80.

45 Grizle JE, Starmer CF, Koch GG. Analysis of categorical data by linear models. Biometrics 1969; *25*: 489-504.

46 Hand DJ, Taylor CC. Multivariate analysis of variance and repeated measures. A practical approach for behavioural scientists. London: Chapman and Hall, 1987.

47 Halford TR. Life-table with concomitant information. Biometrics 1976; *32*: 587-97.

48 Harter HL. Critical values for Ducan's new multiple range test. Biometrics 1960; *16*: 671-85.

49 Harris EK, Albert A. Survivorship analysis for clinical studies. New York: Marcel Dekker, 1991.

50 Hauck WW, Anderson S. A proposal for interpreting and reporting negative studies. Statistics in Medicine 1986; *5*: 203-42.

51 Hills M, Armitage P. The two-period cross-over clinical trial. Br J Clin Pharmacol 1979; *8*: 7-20.

52 Hollander M. Rank tests for randomized blocks when the alternatives have an a priori ordering. Ann Math Statist 1967; *38*: 867-77.

53 House DE. A nonparametric version of William's test for a randomized block design. Biometrics 1986; *42*: 187-90.

54 Huitema BE. The analysis of covariance and alternatives. New York: John Wiley and Sons, 1980.

55 Jenicek M. Méta-analyses en médecine. Evaluation et synthèse de l'information clinique et épidémiologique. Paris: Edisem, St-Hyacinthe, Maloine, 1984.

56 Jenicek M. Meta-analysis in medicine. Where we are and where we want to go. J Clin Epidemiol 1989; *42*: 35-44.

57 Kaiser L. Adjusting for baseline: change or percentage change? Statistics in Medicine 1989; *8*: 1183-90.

58 Kaplan EL, Meier P. Non-parametric estimation from incomplete observations. J Amer Statist Assoc 1958; *53*: 457-81.

59 Kastenbaum MA. A note on the additive partitioning of chi-square in contingency tables. Biometrics 1960; *16*: 416-22.

60 Kenward MG. A method for comparing profiles of repeated measurements. Appl Statist 1987; *36*: 296-308.

61 Keselman HJ, Keselman JC. The analysis of repeated measure designs in medical research. Statistics in Medicine 1984; *3*: 185-95.

62 Klein DF, Ross DC, Feldman S. Analysis and display of psychopharmacological data. J Psychiat Res 1975; *12*: 125-47.

63 Koch GG. Some aspects of the statistical analysis of "split-plot" experiments in completely randomized layouts. Amer Statist Assoc J 1969; *64*: 485-505.

64 Koch GG. The use of non-parametric methods in the statistical analysis of the two-period change-over design. Biometrics 1972; *28*: 577-84.

65 Kock GG, Landis JR, Freeman JL, Freeman DH, Lehnen RG. A general methodology for the analysis of experiments with repeated measurements of categorical data. Biometrics 1977; *33*: 133-58.

66 Kowalski CJ. A commentary on the use of multivariate statistical methods in anthropometric research. Amer J Phys Anthrop 1972; *32*: 119-32.

67 Krauth J. A locally most powerful tied-rank test in a Wilcoxon situation. Ann Math Stat 1971; *42*: 1949-56.

68 Lee J. A note on the comparison of group means based on repeated measurements of the same subject. J Chronic Dis 1980; *33*: 673-5.

69 Lellouch J, Schwartz D. Association de deux variables en tenant compte d'une troi-sième (variables qualificatives). Rev Stat Appliq 1961; *9*: 89-102.

70 Mack GA, Skillings JH. A Friedman-type rank test for main effects in a two-factor ANOVA. J Amer Statist Assoc 1980; *75*: 947-51.

71 Mantel N. Chi-square tests with one degree of freedom: extension of the Mantel-Haenzel procedure. J Amer Statis Assoc 1963; *58*: 690-700.

72 Mantel N. Evaluation of survival data and two new rank order statistics arising in its consideration. Cancer Chemother Reports 1966; *50*: 163-70.

73 Marcus R. The power of some tests of the equality of normal means against an ordered alternative. Biometrika 1976; *63*: 177-83.

74 McHugh R, Matts J. Post-stratification in the randomized clinical trial. Biometrics 1983; *39*: 217-25.

75 Mehta CR, Patel N. A network algorithm for performing Fisher's exact test in r x c contingency tables. J Amer Stat Assoc 1983; *78*: 427-34.

76 Miller RG Jr. Simultaneous statistical inference. New York: McGraw-Hill, 1966.

77 Modd AM. On the asymptotic efficiency of certain non-parametric two sample tests. Ann Math Statist 1954; *25*: 514-22.

78 Mudholkar GS, McDermott MP. A class of tests for equality of ordered means. Biometrika 1989; *76*: 161-8.

79 O'Neill R, Wetherill GB. The present state of multiple comparison methods. J R Statist Soc 1971; *33*: 218-50.

80 Overall JE. General linear model analysis of variance. In: Levine J, ed. Coordinating cli-nical trials in psychopharmacology. Rockville: NIMH, 1979.

81 Pagano M, Halvorsen KT. An algorithm for finding the exact significance levels of r x c contingency tables. J Amer Stat Assoc 1981; *76*: 931-4.

82 Pearson ES, Please NW. Relation between the shape of population distribution and the robustness of four simple test statistics. Biometrika 1975; *62*: 223-41.

83 Permutt T. Testing for imbalance of covariates in controlled experiments. Statistics in Medicine 1990; *9*: 1455-62.

84 Peto R, Pike MC, Armitage P et al. Design and analysis of randomized clinical trials requiring prolonged observation of each patient. I. Introduction and design. Br J Cancer 1977; *35*: 1-39.

85 Philips JPN. More mistakes about interactions. Br J Soc Clin Psychol 1980; *19*: 163-5.

86 Pitman EJG. Significance tests which may be applied to samples from any populations. J R Statist Soc (series B) 1937; *4*: 119-30.

87 Pocock SJ, Geller NL, Tsiatis AA. The analysis of multiple endpoints in clinical trials. Biometrics 1987; *43*: 487-98.

88 Prescott P. Comparison of tests for normality using stylized sensitivity surfaces. Biometrika 1976; *63*: 283-9.

89 Quade D. Rank analysis of covariance. J Amer Statist Assoc 1967; *62*: 1187-200.

90 Raz J. Analysis of repeated measurements using nonparametric smoothers and ran-domization tests. Biometrics 1989; *45*: 851-71.

91 Sacks HS, Berrier J, Reitman D et al. Meta-analysis of randomized controlled trials. N Engl J Med 1987; *316*: 450-5.

92 Scheffe H. An analysis of variance for paired comparison. J Amer Statist Assoc 1952; *47*: 381-400.

93 Scheffe H. A method for judging all constraints in the analysis of variance. Biometrika 1953: *40*: 87-104.

94 Scheffe H. The analysis of variance. New York: John Wiley and Sons, 1959.

95 Scheirer CJ, Ray WS, Hare N. The analysis of ranked data derived from completely randomized factorial designs. Biometrics 1976; *32*: 429-34.

96 Schor SS. Fundamentals of biostatistics. New York: GP Putnam's Sons, 1968: 75-6.

97 Schuirmann DJ. A comparison of two one-sided tests procedure and the power approach for assessing the equivalence of average bioavailability. J Pharmacokinet Biopharm 1987; *15*: 657-80.

98 Sen PK. Robust statistical procedures in problems of linear regression with special reference to quantitative bio-assays. I Rev Int Stat Inst 1971; *39*: 21-38.

99 Senn SJ. Covariate imbalance and random allocation in clinical trials. Statistics in Medicine 1989; *8*: 467-75.

100 Shapiro SS, Wilk MB, Chen HJ. A comparative study of various tests for normality. J Am Statist Assoc 1968; *63*: 1343-72.

101 Siegel S. Non-parametric statistics for the behavioural sciences. New York: McGraw-Hill, 1956.

102 Simes RJ. An improved Bonferroni procedure for muliple tests of significance. Biometrika 1986; *73*: 751-4.

103 Sokal RR, Rohlf FJ. Biometry. San Francisco: W H Freeman and Company, 1969.

104 Spriet A, Beiler D. When can "non-significantly different" treatments be considered as "equivalent" ? Br J Clin Pharmac 1979; *7*: 623-4.

105 Spriet A, Dupin-Spriet T. a) Bonne pratique des essais cliniques des médicaments. Bâle: Karger, 1990. b) Good practice of clinical drug trials. Basel: Karger, 1992.

106 Spriet A, Simon P. Clinical trials: rules and errors. In: Human psychopharmacology. Measures and methods. Vol 2. Hindmarch I, Stonier P, eds. New-York: John Wiley and Sons, 1989: 251-69.

107 Stablein DM, Carter WH, Novack JW. Analysis of survival data using non proportional hazard functions. Controlled Clinical Trials 1981; *2*: 149-59.

108 Stucky W, Vollmar J. Exact probabilities for tied linear rank tests. J Statist Comput Simul 1976; *5*: 73-81.

109 Tandon PK. Applications of global statistics in analyzing quality of life. Statistics in Medicine 1990; *9*: 819-27.

110 Terry ME. Some rank order tests which are most powerful against specific parametric alternatives. Ann Mathem Statist 1952; *23*: 346-66.

111 Thall PF, Lachin JM. Analysis of recurrent events: nonparametric methods for random-interval count data 1988; *83*: 339-47.

112 Wallenstein S, Fisher AC. The analysis of the two-period repeated measurement cross-over design with application to clinical trials. Biometrics 1977; *33*: 261-9.

113 Welch BL. The generalization of Student's problem when several different population variances are involved. Biometrika 1947; *34*: 28-35.

114 Whitehead J, Jones D. The analysis of sequential clinical trials. Biometrika 1978; *66*: 443-52.

115 Williams DA. A test for differences between treatment means when several dose levels are compared with a zero control. Biometrics 1971; *27*: 103-17.

116 Williams DA. The comparison of several dose levels with a zero control. Biometrics 1972; *28*: 519-31.

117 Winer BJ, Brown DR, Michels KM. Statistical principles in experimental design. 3rd edition. New York: McGraw Hill, 1991.

118 Woolf B. The log-likelihood ratio test (the G-test). Methods and tables for tests of heterogeneity in contingency tables. Ann Human Genetics 1957; *21*: 397-409.

119 Yates F. The analysis of contingency tables with groupings based on quantitative characters. Biometrika 1948; *35*: 176-81.

16 - Interim analyses

SUMMARY

It is possible to analyze preliminary results if special precautions are taken (protection of the secret randomization, limited circulation of the results, transparency in the final study report). Group 1 sequential analysis have the objective of stopping the trial as soon as the difference becomes significant. They require intermediate and terminal levels of significance taking the repetition of tests into account. Other methods aim to stop the trial if the hope of obtaining a significant difference becomes too small. Lastly, it is possible to readjust the calculation of the sample size if it has been underestimated.

Continuous sequential methods allow repeated statistical comparison as the trial proceeds after each case (or pair of cases) which means that the trial can be stopped as soon as enough data have been collected to reject one of the hypothesis formulated (null or alternative hypotheses). Closed sequential tests entail termination of a trial once a predetermined maximum number of patients has been enlisted.

Several types of sequential tests are available including sequential tests for the number of preferences between two treatments (in paired subjects or in a within-patient, crossover trial), tests for analyzing differences between paired Gaussian variables, sequential methods for analysis of variance, and non-parametric sequential methods. Sequential tests generally enable a conclusion to be reached with fewer subjects but they may require difficult pairing and they can only be used for treatments of short duration compared to the interval between subject admissions to the trial.
Lastly, sequential methods raise the psychological issue of pursuing a trial when the intermediate results seem to indicate that one treatment is better than another, even though such preliminary results may not be conclusive.

It is not possible to perform repeated analyses of a trial with an increasing number of cases without taking certain precautions. Indeed, the classical theory of tests cannot be applied in this case, since comparisons are not independent and the level of probability calculated would be incorrect.

Thus, a strategy of intermediate analysis is necessary, according to the objectives of this analysis (figure 1). Indeed, there are many methods available depending on:
- if the intermediate analysis is planned in advance or is decided upon due to unforseen circumstances,
- if the objective of the intermediate analysis is to stop the trial if there are sufficient results,
- if the analysis involves cases actually underway or only completed cases,
- whether *groups* of cases are analyzed, or if a test is repeated after *each* case (this latter point will be considered at the end of the chapter under the heading "continuous sequential analysis"),
- the methods used to correct the level of significance of tests.

1. GENERAL PRINCIPLES

To be credible, intermediate analyses must obey strict rules, preferably defined in written procedures, making it possible to verify a posteriori that the strategy was adhered to.

The following few principles apply in all cases.

1.1. Conditions

Intermediate analysis assumes that the first results predict the last ones. This condition is not fulfilled if, for the disorder under study, there is a chronological effect, especially a seasonal one, or if, in a long-term follow-up, one treatment is better than the other at the beginning of the trial but not at the end.

1.2. Decisions

Insofar as possible, an intermediate analysis particularly with stopping rules must be planned in advance, and in this case, it must be stipulated in the protocol. If the analysis, planned in the protocol, is modified, for whatever reason, the decision-making process must at least have been planned (who can take this initiative and who verifies it?).

1.3. Decoding

The intermediate analysis leads to decoding of the randomization procedure. Access to the code, which must be protected, requires particular precautions to avoid "leaks" outside of the persons responsible for analyzing and interpreting the results, and to avoid decoding the treatments not yet analyzed (cases in progress), cases not yet ready for analysis, or treatments not yet attributed.

1.4. Limited circulation

Circulation of the results of the intermediate analysis must be strictly limited to the person responsible for decisions made (in particular rules on stopping the trial). The results must not be known by the investigators unless the decision to stop the trial is made. Indeed, this would risk discouraging them from continuing the trial while the results are still insufficient.

1.5. Corrected data

The intermediate analysis must involve data which have been thoroughly verified and corrected, even if this only concerns part of the elements available as of the day the analysis is made. Indeed, there is a risk that correction may lead to changes in the assessment of cases, which can lead to change the results.

1.6. Final analysis

The final analysis must take the intermediate analysis into account. In particular, the final test must have a corrected level of significance, and the confidence interval must be adapted to the intermediate analyses, which has the effect of widening it (11, 19, 30).

1.7. Transparency

The intermediate analysis must be "transparent", even if its results are not circulated, and it must be clearly visible along with all its consequences in the final trial report.

1.8. Transparency in the product file

If a trial is stopped early due to intermediate results, its results must be clearly visible in the product file, so as not to select more or less subconsciously trials that are favorable to the hypothesis defended.

2. PLANNED INTERMEDIATE ANALYSIS

A planned intermediate analysis must be listed in the study protocol with a certain number of information: number and chronology of analyses planned, statistical method used, rules on decision-making (in particular on stopping the trial in light of the results), and consequences on the final analysis, on the calculation of the sample size, (which should be increased in comparisons to a normal analysis to take any loss of power into account), and interpretation of all the results.
A large number of methods are available, to answer different questions.

2.1. Methods intended to stop the trial as soon as the difference is significant: "Are intermediate results sufficient to draw conclusions ?"

To reach this objective, so-called "group sequential analysis" is used. The principle involved here is simple: intermediate analyses with a reduced level of significance are performed and the final test is corrected according to these analyses. The choice of intermediate and final levels of significance offers several possibilities :

- Pocock's technique (26, 27) consists of making repeated tests with an equal level of significance, taking into account the repetition, including the final test (for example, three tests with $\alpha = 0.022$ for an overall probability of a type I error equal to 5%).
The advantage of this method is that it enables early detection of a larger difference than planned and prevents the continuation of a trial while the response is already known.
The disadvantage is that it decreases the sensitivity of the final test, and if the intermediate results have not made it possible to draw conclusions, the sensitivity of the comparison is decreased. It therefore must be compensated for by making a marked increase in the sample size.

- In Peto's method (25), intermediate tests are run with a very low level of significance (for example, 0.001), which has little impact on the level of significance of the final test. This method only enables detection of very large differences (very underestimated at the start), which occurs rarely.

- O'Brien and Fleming's method (24) is an intermediate between the previous two methods: the first test is run with a very low level of significance, the second with a level slightly higher, and at the end the level of significance of the final test must be reduced slightly (for example for three tests $\alpha = 0.05$; $\alpha = 0.014$; α 0.045, for a 5% overall level of significance).

- Other approaches are possible, with different intermediate levels of significance (16, 20) or with flexible levels of significance making it possible to "spend" the amount of type I error available (21, 22).

- Generally, to conserve the same level of type I error, the sample size of the trial (with the hypothesis that it will continue to the end) must be increased in a proportion which is a function of the method and in relation to the number of intermediate tests (17).

Other methods allow intermediate analyses to be made with the same principle but for studies on survival with prolonged periods of treatment: the tests are run in the same patients, with increasing durations of treatment (5, 7).

It has been pointed out that the choice of one rule or another is not without influence on the result: the same data can lead to different conclusions depending on the method chosen. One thus should clearly understand the advantages and disadvantages of each technique before choosing one.

2.2. Methods intended to stop a trial if the hope of obtaining a significant difference becomes too small.

The methods used for this purpose are of an entirely different type: they consist, taking into account the results acquired during the trial, of estimating the chances of obtaining a satisfactory response to the final analysis. If these chances are satisfactory, the trial is continued, if not the trial is abandoned: "hopeless". Here too, there are several possible techniques:

- A one-tailed test in the direction opposite of the expected favorable result: in practice, with half-sample-size, a "placebo superior to active drug difference" (even if not significant) makes it very unlikely to obtain a significant result with a double sample size. This very simple method results in very little loss of power (less than 1%). If the test is done even earlier, with one-third of expected sample size, there is a loss of power of about 5%. This method is applicable in placebo-controlled trials where a one-tailed test is planned with a binary response.

- Calculation of the probability of obtaining a significant result considering the intermediate results (conditional probability) can be used (12, 14, 15, 18, 36). If the trial is stopped for this reason, it will not be used to prove a difference: the probability associated with the final test will not be distorted and it thus is not necessary to adjust the level of significance. This approach can be improved by taking the following into account:
• data prior to the trial, which the intermediate results have just confirmed or disproved, and which are taken into consideration in a "Bayesian" probability for the final results (17, 37);
• the cost or the loss in the event of negative results, in a "decisional" strategy (8), enabling a cost/benefit analysis considering both economic evidence, prior information, and intermediate results;
• by combining: a method for stopping the trial if the chances of obtaining favorable results are too small, and a method for stopping if the intermediate results are very favorable (36).

2.3. Analysis intended to readjust the final sample size of the trial

With this approach, the objective is not to decrease the sample size but rather to increase it, in the event that intermediate results demonstrate an underestimation of the initial sample size. The analysis then consists of re-estimating the variance of the response with intermediate data, and taking it into account for the re-estimation of the sample size. This re-estimation should only be made in the direction of an increase and never in the direction of a decrease. Under these conditions, the intermediate analysis does not include rules for stopping the trial, and does not distort the level of significance of the final test. For a double-blind trial, this analysis must be made without decoding if possible, focusing the analysis on the results, with all groups combined. The risk of a negative study by under-estimating the size of the sample is considerably reduced (38).

3. UNPLANNED INTERMEDIATE ANALYSIS

Even when the intermediate analysis is not stipulated in the protocol, there are cases where it becomes necessary. To make this possible, while at the same time avoiding chaotic and uncontrolled analyses, precise rules are necessary.

3.1. Justification

The reasons which lead to analyze the results of an uncompleted trial may be as follows:

- Alarming information on the tolerability of the test drugs.
The expected benefit/risk ratio of the new treatment can thus have sharply deteriorated. Tolerability below what was expected can only be compensated for by better than expected efficacy. An intermediate analysis of efficacy is thus useful in deciding whether to stop or to continue the development program.

- An independent unfavorable result of efficacy.
A program of drug development always includes several trials with different durations and sample sizes. It is not rare that the results of one or more completed trials again question the need for continuing the trials in progress, or in limiting the indications of the drug under study. Before a vital decision on the product is made, examination of intermediate results of a prolonged trial is necessary since it is not possible to wait for definitive results which will come much later on. There is also an ethical consideration which consists of assessing the judgment of continuing a trial when another trial has yielded very unfavorable results.

- Economic reasons.
The value of a program may be called into question by an advance made by a competitor, or by a product licensing-out project. Here too, the decision to stop or to continue the program can be influenced by the available results of uncompleted trials whose completion cannot be waited for.

- Bad reasons.
Among all the reasons which lead the organizers of a trial to examine its results during the trial, some are not all equally valid: curiosity, the need to be reassured, the search of esteem by announcing results in a preliminary presentation, the unwise listing of a communication at a congress, or even the temptation of providing the most favorable results possible by stopping trials which are yielding negative results at the most "opportune" moment. To avoid unavowable reasons, concealed behind pseudo-rationales, safeguards are necessary.

3.2. Decisions

If not stipulated in the protocol, the decision to make an intermediate analysis can be made with safeguards making it possible to avoid having unjustifiable reasons lead to chaotic pirated analyses. A written procedure is necessary specifying <u>who</u> has the right to make the decision, which <u>document</u> must be signed and by whom, and in which form the <u>justification</u> must be formulated and written. Furthermore, before making the analysis, the decision on which method will be used must be made and how it will be taken into account in the final analysis. It must be specified as to who will know of the existence of the analysis and its results, to limit their circulation if a decision to stop the trial is not made. Lastly, assurance must be made that the intermediate analsysis will be mentioned in the final trial report.

3.3. Consequences

- If the analysis of partial results leads to stopping of the trial, obviously the investigators must be notified, as well as all other persons working on

Figure 1
Intermediate analysis

Planned ?
- objective
- number
- chronology of events or amount of information
- type of analysis

no

Unplanned:
- justify (unplanned event)
- decide as to who decides ? choice of the method and circulation of results

yes

Analysis of partial results

Group sequential analysis

Stochastic discontinuation

Internal pilot study

Analysis of partial results

Termination

Termination (conclusive result)

Termination (unfavourable trend unlikely to be reversed)

Increase N: σ^2 underestimated, placebo effect underestimated, frequency of events overestimated

Continuation (α must be corrected)

Continuation (α must be corrected)

Continuation (loss of power)

Continuation (α must be corrected)

FINAL ANALYSIS MENTIONING THE INTERMEDIATE ANALYSES

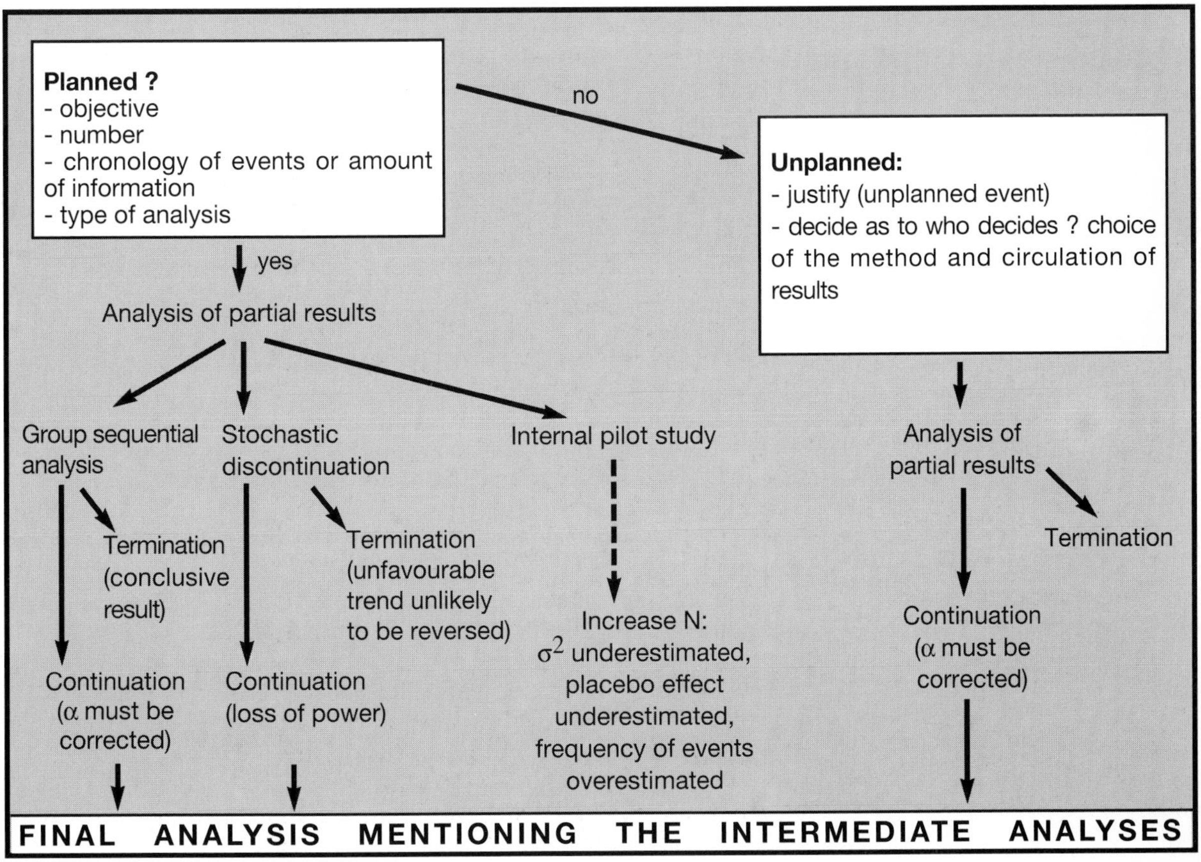

the trial. In particular, this result must be mentioned in the product file if it is submitted to drug registration authorities at some later date.

- If the intermediate analysis leads to continue the trial to its planned completion, this must be taken into account in the final analysis by adjusting the level of significance (4), so that it is not distorted by an intermediate analysis, and to discuss its consequences.

4. CONTINUOUS SEQUENTIAL ANALYSIS

Sequential analysis is the extreme form of intermediate analyses: the test is repeated with each case or each pair of cases.

• The principle of the method may be summed up as follows:

- a choice must be made between a null hypothesis (no difference between the results of the treatments compared) and an alternative hypothesis (minimum difference Δ we wish to demonstrate with a reasonable chance).

- we define the acceptable probability for rejecting the null hypothesis if it is true (α) and rejecting the alternative hypothesis if it is true (β);

- with each new case (or pair of cases, according to the method used), we must calculate a new value for the test. This value is then compared to a maximum and a minimum value determined in advance depending on α, β and Δ. If the maximum value is exceeded, the null hypothesis is rejected; if the value is lower than the minimum value, the alternative hypothesis is rejected. This means that the treatment results are equivalent within Δ. In both cases, the trial must be stopped;

- as long as the value of the test remains within these two limits, we will continue to enlist subjects.

To avoid prolonging the trial unduly (by bad luck), one should, whenever possible, limit the *maximum* number of cases, for which the alternative hypothesis will be rejected even if the value of the test does not fall beyond the predefined limits. Thus we perform a closed sequential test (as opposed to the *open* test, which can in theory last a very long time, although with an increasingly low probability of crossing the boundaries of maximum and minimum values).

• The principal sequential tests than can be used in clinical trials are shown in table 1. *Closed sequential tests* cannot be used for certain designs, thus restricting their use.

Lastly, other sequential methods more logically fall within the scope of "decisional" methods described in another chapter.

Table I Sequential tests

Situations	Tests	References	Remarks
Counting of preferences for one of two treatments (matched pairs of within-patient crossover trial). Pairs without a preference ties are disregarded.	One or two-tailed open or closed binomial sequential test. The limits of closed tests have been tabulated only for usual cases. In other circumstances, the approximative method described by Armitage may be used (1, 2).	(1, 2, 10, 13)	This is the most classical method and it consists of plotting the number of cases on the x-axis and the difference in the number of preference for one or the other of the treatments on the y-axis. The approximate boundaries are straight lines; the exact boundaries have been calculated for some values of the alternate hypothesis and some probabilities α and β.
Dichotomous criterion: counting successes and failures for two treatments (paired cases or within-patient crossover trial)	Simon, Weiss and Hoel's method.	(35)	"Three hypotheses model". This method uses all pairs including those for which no preference is expressed.
Gaussian variables: two treatments (paired cases or within-patient trial).	Sequential test: open or closed, one or two-tailed sequential t test (sequential equivalent of the paired t test). For the closed test, an approximation is used	(23, 32, 33) (1) (2)	The boundaries of this tests may be found in tables (6) but complex interpolations are required. An easier to use approximation has been described (31). If the variances are expected to be different, see (29)
Gaussian variables (≥ 2 treatments), parallel groups.	One-way sequential analysis of variance.	(28)	• This test is recalculated for each subject enlisted per treatment • No closed version exists for this test.
Gaussian variables (≥ 2 treatments), within-subject or paired data	Sequential analysis of variance (randomized blocks)	(28)	• At each step a decision is taken as to whether to stop the trial or add another "block" (pair of cases or one subject in a within-patient trial). • No closed version exists for this test.

4.1. Advantages

The advantage of a sequential test is that one is able to reach a conclusion with fewer subjects, on the *average,* than are required for a classical test.

In reality, however, the number of subjects that have to be treated before reaching a conclusion is sometimes higher than with a classical method. The sample size needed cannot be determined but becomes a random variable, for which one can only predict the average size. Reaching a conclusion with fewer participants exposed to risk offers an ethical advantage which is often put forward as an argument to promote the use of sequential methods. During the trial fewer patients need to receive the treatment which proves the least effective. The more speedily the result of the comparison is known, the sooner future patients can benefit from it.

4.2. Disadvantages

• Many sequential methods require the comparison of subjects in pairs, and this means forming comparable pairs of subjects based upon those characteristics liable to influence the results. The practical problems involved in *pairing* the subjects tend to delay rather than to hasten the trial (if each patient has to wait until he finds the *right "match"*).

• In a sequential test, each case (or pair) should ideally be completed before others can be admitted to the trial. The observation period for each patient must therefore be *short in comparison to the interval between subjects being admitted to the trial.*

• Lastly, as for any intermediate analysis, it may be difficult from a psychological point of view, to continue prescribing a treatment which "appears" the least effective on the basis of intermediate results which are not conclusive and therefore mandate continuing the trial.

References

1 Armitage P. Restricted sequential procedures. Biometrika 1957; *44*: 9-26.

2 Armitage P. Sequential medical trials. 2nd edition. Oxford: Blackwell Scientific Publications, 1975.

3 Armitage P. Interim analysis in clinical trials. Statistics in Medicine 1991; *10*: 925-37.

4 Armitage P, McPherson CK, Rowe BC. Repeated significance tests on accumulating data. J R Statistic Soc A 1969; *132*: 235-44.

5 Armitage P, Stratton IM, Worthington HV. Repeated significance tests for clinical trials with a fixed number of patients and variable follow-up. Biometrics 1985; *41*: 353-9.

6 Arnold KJ. Tables to facilitate sequential tests. Applied Math; *ser. n° 7*. National Bureau of Standards. US Government Printing Office, Washington, 1951.

7 Benichou J, Chastang Cl. Analyse séquentielle des essais thérapeutiques randomisés dont le critère de jugement est la survie. Utilisation du test triangulaire. Thérapie 1987; *42*: 295-9.

8 Berry DA, Ho CH. One-sided sequential stopping boundaries for clinical trials: a decision-theoretic approach. Biometrics 1988; *44*: 219-27.

9 Bristol DR. A one-sided interim analysis with binary outcomes. Controlled Clinical Trials 1988; *9*: 206-11.

10 Bross I. Sequential medical plans. Biometrics 1952; *8*: 188-205.

11 Chang MN. Confidence intervals for a normal mean following a group sequential test. Biometrics 1989; *45*: 247-54.

12 Chi PY, Bristol DR, Castellana JV. A clinical trial with an interim analysis. Statistics in Medicine 1986; *5*: 387-92.

13 Choi SC. Truncated sequential designs for clinical trials based on Markov chains. Biometrics 1968; *24*: 159-68.

14 Choi SC, Pepple PA. Monitoring clinical trials based on predictive probability of significance. Biometrics 1989; *45*: 317-23.

15 Choi SC, Smith PJ, Becker DP. Early decision in clinical trials when the treatment differences are small. Experience of a controlled clinical trial in head trauma. Controlled Clinical Trials 1986; *6*: 280-8.

16 Falissard B, Lellouch J. Some extensions to a new approach for interim analysis in clinical trials. Statistics in Medicine 1991; *10*: 949-57.

17 Geller NL, Pocock SJ. Interim analysis in randomized clinical trials: ramifications and guidelines for practitioners. Biometrics 1987; *43*: 213-23.

18 Halperin M, Lan KK, Ware JH, Johnson NJ, DeMets DL. An aid to data monitoring in long-term clinical trials. Controlled Clinical Trials 1982; *3*: 311-23.

19 Jennison C, Turnbull BW. Interim analyses: the repeated confidence interval approach. J R Statist Soc B 1989; *51*: 305-61.

20 Koepke W. Analyses of group sequential clinical trials. Controlled Clinical Trials 1989; *10*: 222S-30S.

21 Kim K, DeMets DL. Designs and analysis of group sequential tests based on the type I error spending rats function. Biometrika 1987; *74*: 149-54.

22 Lan KKG, DeMets DL. Discrete sequential boundaries for clinical trials. Biometrika 1983; *70*: 659-63.

23 Myers MH, Schneiderman MA, Armitage P. Boundaries for closed (wedge) sequential t-test plans. Biometrika 1963; *53*: 431-7.

24 O'Brien PC, Fleming TR. A multiple testing procedure for clinical trials. Biometrics 1979; *35*: 549-56.

25 Peto R, Pike MC, Armitage P et al. Design and analysis of randomized clinical trials requiring prolonged observation of each patient. I. Introduction and design. Br J Cancer 1976; *34*: 585-612. II. Analysis and examples. Br J Cancer 1977; *35*: 1-39.

26 Pocock SJ. Group sequential methods in the design and analysis of clinical trials. Biometrika 1977; *64*: 191-9.

27 Pocock SJ, Hughes MD. Practical problems in interim analyses, with particular regard to estimation. Controlled Clinical Trials 1989; *10*: 209S-21S.

28 Ray WD. Sequential analysis applied to certain experimental designs in the analysis of variance. Biometrika 1956; *43*: 388-403.

29 Robbins H, Simons G, Starr N. A sequential analogue of the Behrens-Fisher problem. Ann Math Statist 1967; *38*: 1384-91.

30 Rosner GL, Tsiatis AA. Exact confidence intervals following a group sequential trial: a comparison of methods. Biometrika 1988; *75*: 723-9.

31 Rushtons S. On a sequential t-test. Biometrika 1952; *37*: 326-33.

32 Schneiderman MA, Armitage P. A family of closed sequential procedures. Biometrika 1962; *49*: 41-56.

33 Schneiderman MA, Armitage P. Closed sequential t-test. Biometrika 1962; *49*: 359-66.

34 Schultz JR, Elfring GL. Group sequential rank sum test. 27th Annual Princeton Conference, Princeton NJ. Dec 3, 1971.

35 Simon R, Weiss GH, Hoel DG. Sequential analysis of binomial clinical trials. Biometrika 1975; *62*: 195-200.

36 Ware JH, Muller JE, Braunwald E. The futility index. An approach to the cost-effective termination of randomized clinical trials. Amer J Med 1985; *78*: 635-43.

37 Whitehead J. Four problems with group sequential methods. Controlled Clinical Trials 1991; *12*: 340-4.

38 Wittes J, Brittain E. The role of internal pilot studies in increasing the efficiency of clinical trials. Statistics in Medicine 1990; *9*: 65-72.

17 - Exploratory analyses

SUMMARY

The analysis of secondary criteria carries less weight than that of the principal criterion. If planned in the protocol before the trial begins, it represents an intermediate state between confirmatory and exploratory analyses. However, it always requires cautious interpretation.

The analysis of subgroups must avoid circular reasoning. A strategy for analysis is proposed in the following discussion.

After the efficacy of a drug has been demonstrated in a controlled trial, it may be of interest to define a "responder" and "non-responder" profile to determine therapeutic indications more precisely. This can be accomplished through "predictive analysis" in which the initial pretreatment characteristics of subjects for whom treatment has resulted in either satisfactory or unsatisfactory results is compared. This analysis may subsequently permit a more discriminating choice between the treatments considered (but only these) administered under the same conditions for any future given patient.

Predictive variables include the subjects' demographic characteristics, physiology, psychology, symptoms or the nosological category.

Multivariate statistical methods may be used: in particular, discriminant functions (if the response to treatment can be expressed dichotomously) or multiple regression (if the response is expressed quantitatively, as for example with improvement in a test score).

The results of such studies must be validated by verifying their predictive value in subjects other than those who served to establish the algorithms for predicting response.

The principle involved in the confirmatory statistical test is based on calculating probabilities, which is accurate if the study data are used only once and if it answers a question formulated a priori. This is why the protocol of a comparative trial is built to answer only a simple main question.

In practice, the information provided by the trial greatly surpasses the question formulated and so cannot be overlooked. Such information does not enable firm conclusions to be drawn: it is exploratory. Three such categories can be defined:
- secondary criteria planned in the protocol,
- analysis into subgroups,
- predictive retrospective analysis.

1. ACCESSORY CRITERIA PLANNED IN THE PROTOCOL

In addition to the principal criterion used in the confirmatory analysis, several other evaluations are often collected:
- a new method of investigation in addition to the classical technique,
- several symptoms measured independently,
- the severity of attacks of disease in addition to their frequency,
- the efficacy-compliance with treatment relationship...

The results of comparison of treatments based on these criteria are less convincing than the principal test. Nonetheless, several factors weigh in the balance of this observation. The conclusions are strengthened if:
- the difference observed with an accessory criterion goes in the same direction as the answer to the principal question,
- all accessory criteria provide concurring and plausible answers,
- the results of statistical tests performed for descriptive purposes yield very small probabilities,
- care is taken to adjust the level of significance for multiple tests.

When the protocol specifies multiple tests and their adjustment, it may be considered that we are in a situation that lies between exploratory and confirmatory analysis (2).

2. ANALYSIS OF SUBGROUPS

Since there may be an unlimited number of subgroups, it is important to have a strategy of analysis to avoid *circular reasoning*: a hypothesis generated in light of the results and confirmed by these same results. Indeed, it is always possible to find, post hoc, subgroups which had a different outcome even by comparing subjects who received the *same* treatment (22).
This strategy may be based on the organization chart presented in figure 1 by answering the following questions (7, 9, 43):

• Can the subgroup under consideration be of clinical interest ?
This may be the case, for example with diabetics or elderly subjects. It generally is not true for left-handed persons, red-haired nearsighted individuals or the total number of persons born under the sign of Virgo or Gemini! (3). In practice, examining the results of a priori non-relevant subgroups must be forbidden.

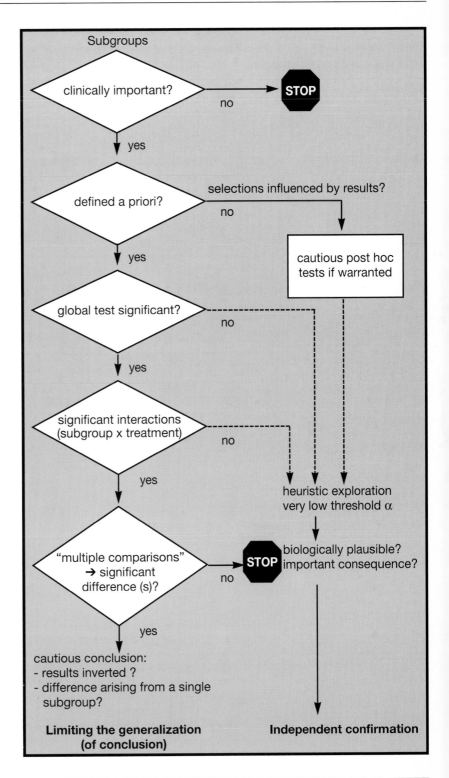

Figure 1
Subgroups: strategy

Subgroups

clinically important? — no → **STOP**

yes

defined a priori? — no → selections influenced by results?

yes

global test significant? — no

yes

significant interactions (subgroup x treatment) — no

yes

cautious post hoc tests if warranted

heuristic exploration very low threshold α

"multiple comparisons" → significant difference (s)? — no → **STOP**

biologically plausible? important consequence?

yes

cautious conclusion:
- results inverted ?
- difference arising from a single subgroup?

Limiting the generalization (of conclusion)

Independent confirmation

• Was the subgroup defined a priori in the protocol (for example, by stratification of randomization), or at least before decoding the results? If the answer is no, once again conclusions must be interpreted cautiously and results communicated with reservation.

• Is the overall test of difference between treatments significant?
If this is the case, analysis of subgroups would result in restrictions in the generalization of results which are nevertheless often acceptable provided they result in being more cautious. Otherwise, only a subgroup that shows a very large difference with a very low and biologically plausible level of significance should be taken into consideration; in any case, it requires independent confirmation.

• In the overall analysis, is the subgroup by treatment interaction significant?
If not, circumspection is necessary.

• Do tests that are separated according to subgroups take into account a correction for multiple comparisons that are not independent (1, 42)?
If not, conclusions should generally be attributed to random variations in results.

Analysis by subgroups is important and interesting but its conclusions must be interpreted with caution. It may lead to restrictions in indications of a treatment, in particular if a subgroup presents results that are reversed in relation to the principal analysis or if it demonstrates a difference arising from a single subgroup. In all other cases, independent confirmation must be sought if the question is of medical interest.

In addition, it is of interest to correct the overestimate of differences observed in extreme subgroups by taking into account overall results of the trial by using a Bayesian method (12).

3. THE PREDICTIVE ANALYSIS

A very important question involves the exact type of patients for whom a treatment can most usefully be prescribed. Obviously, trials for different indications (distinct nosological categories or clinical forms of a disease) and the analysis of subgroups as discussed above can contribute to answering this question. Nevertheless, regardless of the category of subjects one decides to select, no treatment can carry a 100% guarantee of success.

It thus is desirable to have methods that would make it possible to *anticipate* success or failure for a given treatment based on each subject's individual characteristics: demographic, physiological, psychological and pathological. This would enable us to define a *responder* and *non-responder profile*, and thereby use the available treatments as rationally and as efficiently as possible.

The methods used to define such a profile are either retrospective analysis of a clinical trial undertaken for another objective, or the formation of a group of patients treated with this aim, possibly non-comparatively. These methods have been tried mostly for psychotropic drug studies (6, 20, 32), but they may have interesting applications in other areas (25).

It should be noted that the analysis of such studies, which are generally carried out during "phase IV" trials (after a new product has been marketed), is of the "exploratory" type (40). That is, the description of "responder" subgroups and the optimal *a posteriori* combination of the variables describe the responses observed. In such cases, it is rather a question of *generating* hypotheses than of testing them. At a later stage, these hypotheses could be *confirmed* using independent data.

3.1. Sources of data

3.1.1. The non-comparative predictive study

In this type of study, the same treatment is administered to all the subjects and the results are observed. The aim is not to evaluate the efficacy of the treatment (which could only be validly assessed by a comparative trial), but simply to compare the *initial* features of the "responders" (subjects for whom satisfactory results have been obtained) and the "non-responders" (insufficient results). Later, should the prediction prove valid, the treatment may ultimately be administered only to potential responders if their "profile" is easily recognizable. Studies of this type have been published with reference to treatments for depression such as electroconvulsive therapy (10, 17, 18) or amitriptyline (19, 29) or nortriptyline (8). The results of such prediction studies are obviously applicable only to the same type of patient receiving the same treatment under the same conditions.

3.1.2. The predictive analysis of a comparative trial

Such a trial is designed to compare two or more treatments allocated randomly to the patients selected for the study, as in all comparative studies. However, it also includes the *differential* analysis of the responders and non-responders to each treatment (47). The results of this analysis would then enable selection of the treatment most likely to prove successful for any new patient, according to the initial features of the subject.

Even if the comparison as a whole shows one of the treatments to be less effective, it need not systematically be rejected since it can still be used for special types of indications in a subgroup of the population included in the study. The choice of a *treatment* based on a prediction trial obviously concerns only the type of patients included in the trial, and only applies to treatments compared in the trial.

Prediction trials that are more or less convincing, comparing two or three treatments, have been published in the comparison of neuroleptics (15, 16, 21, 27), antidepressants (13, 26, 27, 32, 33, 35, 38) or anorectic drugs (46).

3.2. Prediction variables

Ideally, a prediction trial should be designed to record all the initial features of the subjects likely to be in some way related to the outcome of the treatment, before the latter commences. However, it is impossible to be sure a priori which variables will ultimately prove to be relevant. The amount of data that could be collected is unlimited. (Why disregard the color of a subject's eyes, or the age of his parents at his birth?). The choice therefore has to be fairly arbitrary. We have to restrict ourselves to the variables most likely to be of use in the prediction, on the basis of *currently available knowledge* or hypotheses, and which can be formulated with at least some logical basis. A distinction should be made between analyses of the effects of the treatments as a function of a single feature and "multivariate" analyses including several variables.

• To quote one example, many studies have been published on differential analysis of the effects of treatments for depression based on a *single characteristic*. The results of these studies are not always very convincing and are sometimes difficult to interpret. Some of the characteristics include:
- age, sex, ethnic origin (8, 36, 37),
- symptomatology (14, 30, 35),
- response to previous treatments (28) or to an initial test dose (24),
- a biological criterion (4, 5, 11, 23, 39, 45).

• True responder profile studies take several features into consideration simultaneously (6):
- demographic data, personality,
- personal and family history, nosological classification,
- course of illness, symptomatology,
- laboratory tests in some cases.

3.3. Statistical methods

There are various *"multidimensional" or "multivariate" statistical* techniques available for studying several prediction variables *simultaneously*.

3.3.1. Qualitative criterion

If the feature to be predicted is a qualitative responder-non-responder classification, a *discriminant function* for the sample studied which is the optimal combination of "predictor" variables, can be defined. This function, when applied to a given individual, will make it possible to classify him as a presumed responder or non-responder. The simplest form of discriminant function is the *linear* discriminant function for distinguishing *two* groups. It is established by determining a formula for the sum of the weighted prediction variables which gives the best discrimination (above a given threshold value a subject will be classified as a responder, and below this value as a non-responder). Somewhat more complicated forms of discriminant functions can also be used. These may involve one of the following:

• a *non-linear* combination of variables (for example, calculating the function using the values of the variables and their squares simultaneously);

• more than two groups (for example, very good, fairly good and poor responders);

• techniques whereby the variables are accepted one after the other, and "added" to previously accepted variables in order of supplementary discriminating power until the separation between the groups is no longer significantly improved (*"stepwise"* discriminant analysis). It should be noted that in all the multivariate methods, the importance given to the variables does not reflect their relation with the result but their additional predictive value once the "redundancy" of the other variables has been eliminated;

• a priori probabilities and/or "costs" (i.e. broad sense: quantified disavantage) of prediction errors.

3.3.2. Quantitative criterion

If the criterion that we wish to predict is quantified (for example the predicted improvement of a score on a rating scale), a *multiple regression* method (10, 17, 34) may be used. This procedure entails calculating the best weighted combination of variables whose value is a predictable improvement score.

Besides the linear multiple regression, there are also non-linear regression models (polynomials) and *"stepwise"* methods by which a few of the most "predictive variables" can be selected. General predictive variables are first defined, followed by specific predictors for each treatment. The latter are calculated taking into account the general predictive variables (16).

For a new subject to be treated, a function for each of the treatments is calculated on the basis of the subject's particular features and the weighting factors obtained from previous data. This function enables us to choose the treatment most likely to prove successful.

For prediction purposes, correspondence factorial analysis has been advocated (25, 44). This procedure entails division of quantitative variables into classes, whereby the subjects and the features can be represented in the same coordinate system, and possibly divided into more or less well-defined subgroups. Automatic classification methods can also be used (41).

3.3.3. Validation

When the algorithm (formula for calculation of a discriminant function or a multiple regression) has been established, it can be applied in an attempt to predict the result of a treatment before prescribing it for a new patient (this calculation formula involves the subject's individual features and weighting coefficients obtained from preliminary trial data). The procedure is *"validated"* if the prediction proves accurate more often than would be likely by mere chance. This validation can be achieved by several methods:

• the algorithm can be applied to a new patient population which includes none of the subjects originally used to establish the algorithm (31);

• the original sample of patients can be divided (randomly) into two subgroups, one used to define the algorithm, the other to validate it;

• using a sample of n cases, defining n times a prediction function on n-1 subjects (a different subject is removed from the sample each time) and applying it each time to the nth case, a method derived from statistical techniques known as the "Jackknife" (16).

Any unexpected hypothesis generated by a prediction study must be confirmed by independent data.

4. RE-EXAMINATION OF "SURPRISING" RESULTS

4.1. Circumstances

The results of a clinical trial may be disappointing from the sponsor's stand-point or from that of the advocates of treatment for which the conclusions prove to be unfavorable. Moreover, these results may be unexpected, hard to believe, "too good to be true", or contradict those from other studies.

Although the results a priori are true if the trial has been designed and conducted correctly, doubt may be justified and opens the door to possible reexamination in the following cases:
- the placebo proves as effective or even more so than the active drug contrary to the entire product clinical file,
- the dose-response relationship is not monotonous (the effect increases as a function of the dose and then decreases), contrary to other clinical and pharmacological results,

- a sustained release formulation has effects that last no longer than an ordinary formulation, contrary to other data,
- etc.

Nonetheless, one should be careful not to adopt the attitude whereby only unfavorable results would arouse doubt. This could distort conclusions of a clinical file.

4.2. Possible explanations

All sorts of abnormalities may account for an erroneous result: in the design of the trial, in data collected, in the analysis of results and lastly, chance.

4.2.1. Error in design

It is not a rare occurrence that, in light of the results, regret is expressed with regard to options chosen in the protocol: choice of doses, choice of the comparator, non-centralized or non-stratified randomization, choice of an unconventional criterion of response, an insufficient washout period, a treatment period that is too short, non-standardized concomitant treatments (in case of multiple drug treatments in particular), a sample size that is too small...

When such errors are suggested to explain an unfavorable result, the explanation is only credible if it is consistent with the results of all other trials. It can also represent a simple hypothesis (exploratory analysis) that a new program of trials might demonstrate or refute.

4.2.2. Anomalies involving data

Incidents which have occurred in the observance of the study protocol may distort data. But, here too, explanations can only be provided with reservations, since they are proposed in the light of the results.

- If the double-blind method was not complied with (in particular because the study drugs were not perfectly identical in appearance, so that treatment allocation was biased, or evaluation was distorted because the nature of the treatment was known), it is necessary, first, to describe this anomaly quantitatively and qualitatively after making a thorough investigation. One can then make supplementary exploratory analyses on subsets of cases for which treatments were assigned correctly, if they are numerous enough.

- If it is suspected that seasonal or geographic differences may have introduced bias into the trial, they must be supported by precise data on these factors. They may possibly be taken into account in an exploratory analysis. Any confirmation by independent data will be a welcome event.

- If dissimilar groups are observed, despite correct randomization, these dissimilarities must be investigated. Their extent and their relation to the results must be evaluated. The error that they may have occasioned must be studied. It must be determined whether this is in the same direction and with the same magnitude as the unexpected result observed. Here too, independent confirmation is desirable.

- If it is suspected that unequal compliance with treatment was unfavorable to one of the study drugs, precise data for each subject must be available. An exploratory analysis of the result adjusted according to compliance with therapy can possibly be made. Confirmation by independent data is necessary.
Indeed, compliance with therapy may depend on the result and conversely, and therefore this does not involve a true covariate.

- If the principal criterion of response is the assessment of a symptom for which a fail-safe treatment is planned, a difference in efficacy could have been masked by increased consumption of this drug in the group receiving the least effective treatment. As an exploratory measure, post-stratification by extent of consumption of the symptomatic treatment may be tried, or analysis of a composite index including both the symptom and the alternate treatment. This latter procedure is hazardous. The index is hardly credible unless it is supported by, on one hand, a metrological study of this criterion (sensitivity specificity, and reproducibility) and on the other hand, a new trial taking it as the principal criterion.

- If a labelling error is suspected, for example, complete transposition of treatments, a very careful investigation must be made. This explanation can not be advanced without actual proof. An analysis made after treatments have been corrected will never be very conclusive.

- If laxity in data collection is suspected (rounding-off numbers, a high proportion of missing data...), an unexpected result could thus be explained provided that it is an *attenuation* of differences. This explanation must be supported by an examination of the loss of information, notably its order of magnitude.

- If a malfunction in equipment designed to measure the criterion of response is suspected (for example, inaccurate calibration or increasingly inaccurate measurements), a "correction" in results depending on an estimate of "drift" in measurements may be attempted, but solely as an exploratory measure. Thus it is possible to invalidate the results of the first analysis yet still not obtain entirely convincing data.

4.2.3. Anomalies concerning the analysis

- The analysis as provided for in the protocol may have erroneously used a method that was not very robust, for which conditions of applicability were not adhered to. In this case, the post hoc decision of having recourse to a more suitable method can be justified, provided that one remains within the area of simple techniques, avoiding unconventional transformations, and multiple adjustments. This must be shown in the report. When no precaution is contained in the study protocol, the analysis thus modified is credible especially if it is made after observation of the violations of conditions for its application, but before the method initially planned is used.

- If the method planned for in the protocol is inappropriate, leading to too much lost information (for example transformation of a quantitative variable into classes), use of a more sensitive method is justified as a secondary measure, provided that it is not in flagrant contradiction with the method originally planned.

- The most frequent cases involve interactions which prove to have a greater impact than planned, in particular: a qualitative interaction i.e. center x treatment or subgroup x treatment. A separate exploratory analysis of subsets of cases may prove necessary, but to the detriment of the generalization of results.

4.2.4. Random error

A possible type I error must not be ruled out (a false difference that appears when the treatments are equivalent), or a type II error (a real difference that is concealed by random variations). It is the comparison of results of several trials and the contradiction of results which makes it possible to support this explanation. It is the existence of a type I error notably which justifies the fact that certain drug registration authorities require *two* redundant *placebo-controlled* trials to demonstrate the efficacy of a drug.

4.3. Measures to be taken

In all cases, if an unexpected, untoward or hard-to-believe result is observed, the following measures should be followed:

- Do not try, at all costs, to discredit either this single result or the centers in a multicenter trial whose results are surprising, ("bias by seeking bias"). If a quality audit of the study results in disqualification of part of the results, the trials or centers which contradict them must be validated, using the same auditing procedure, and in any case, conclusions may be drawn only with cautious reservation.

- The proposed explanation must be supported not only with data from the study but also with other known facts on the product, and on the disorder under study. When the stakes are high, it may be necessary to undertake further studies upon completion of this investigation.

- Any post hoc analysis decided upon must be considered as exploratory. It enables the generation of ideas, explanations and hypotheses.

Thus, it is only when the entire file is considered (including any possible meta-analysis of studies with which the protocol is compatible), that contradictory results may be assessed.

References

1 Abt K. Problems of repeated significance testing. Controlled Clinical Trials 1981; *1*: 377-81.

2 Abt K. Planning controlled clinical trials on the basis of descriptive data analysis. Statistics in Medicine 1991; *10*: 777-95.

3 Anonymous. Randomised trial of intravenous streptokinase, oral aspirin, both, or neither among 17 187 cases of suspected acute myocardial infarction ISIS 2. Lancet 1988; *ii*: 350-60.

4 Beckman H, Goodwin FK. Antidepressant response to tricyclics and urinary MHPG in unipolar patients. Arch Gen Psychiatry 1975; *32*: 17-21.

5 Beckman H, Murphy DL. Phenelzine in depressed patients. Effects on urinary MHPG excretion in relation to clinical response. Neuropsychobiology 1977; *3*: 49-55.

6 Bielski RJ, Friedel RO. Prediction of tricyclic antidepressant response. A critical review. Arch Gen Psychiatry 1976; *33*: 1479-89.

7 Bulpitt C.J. Subgroup analysis. Lancet 1988; *ii*: 31-4.

8 Burrows GD, Foenander G, Davies B, Scoggino BA. Rating scales as predictors of response to tricyclic antidepressants. Austr N-Z J Psychiatry 1976; *10*: 53-6.

9 Byar DP. Assessing apparent treatment-covariate interactions in randomized clinical trials. Statistics in Medicine 1985; *4*: 255-63.

10 Carney MWP, Roth M, Garside RF. The diagnosis of depressive syndrome and the prediction of ECT response. Br J Psychiat 1965; *111*: 659-74.

11 Carroll BJ, Feinberg M, Greden JF. A specific laboratory test for the diagnosis of melancholia. Arch Gen Psychiatry 1981; *38*: 15-22.

12 Davis CE, Leffingwell DP. Empirical Bayes estimates of subgroup effects in clinical trials. Controlled Clinical Trials 1990; *11*: 37-42.

13 Finnerty RF, Goldberg HL. Specific response to imipramine and doxepin in psychoneurotic depressed patients with sleep disturbance. J Clin Psychiatry 1981; *42*: 275-9.

14 Garside RF. The comparative value of types of rating scales. Br J Clin Pharm 1976; *suppl*: 61-7.

15 Goldberg SC, Mattson N, Cole JO, Klerman GC. Prediction of improvement in schizophrenia under four phenothiazines. Arch Gen Psychiatry 1967; *16*: 107-17.

16 Goldberg SC, Schooler NR, Hogarty GE, Roper M. Prediction of relapse in schizophrenic outpatients treated by drug and sociotherapy. Arch Gen Psychiatry 1977; *34*: 171-88.

17 Hamilton M, White JM. Factors related to the outcome of depression treated with ECT. J Mental Sciences 1960; *106*: 1031-41.

18 Hamilton M. Prediction of response to ECT in depressive illness. Classification and prediction of outcome of depression. Symposium Schloss Reinhartshausen/Rhein, September 23rd-26th: 1973. Chairman: Angst J. Stuttgart: Schattauer Verlag, 1974.

19 Horden A, Holt NF, Burt CG, Gordon WF. Amitriptyline in depressive states. Br J Psychiatry 1963; *109*: 815-25.

20 Kerr TA, Roth M, Schapara K, Gurney C. The assessment and prediction of outcome in affective disorders. Br J Psychiatry 1972; *121*: 167-74.

21 Klett CJ, Mosely EC. The right drug for the right patient. J Consulting Psychology 1965; *29*: 546-51.

22 Lee KL, McNeer F, Starmer CF et al. Clinical judgment and statistics. Lessons from a simulated randomized trial in coronary artery disease. Circulation 1988; *61*: 508-15.

23 Maas JW, Fawcett JA, Dekirmenjian H. Catecholamine metabolism, depressive illness, and drug response. Arch Gen Psychiatry 1972; *26*: 252-62.

24 May PR, Van Putten T, Yale C et al. Predicting individual responses to drug treatment in schizophrenia: a test dose model. J Nerv Ment Dis 1976; *162*: 177-83.

25 Nakache JP, Lorente P. Multidimensional techniques for the routine assessment of prognosis in patients with acute myocardial infarction. Medinfo 77 IFIP, North-Holland Publishing Company, 1977.

26 Overall JE, Hollister L, Johnson M, Pennington V. Nosology of depression and differential response to drugs. J Amer Med Assoc 1966; *195*: 162-4.

27 Overall JE, Hollister LE, Honigfled G et al. Comparison of acetophenazine with perphenazine in schizophrenics: demonstration of differential effects based on a computer-derived diagnostic model. Clin Pharmacol Ther 1973; *4*: 200-8.

28 Pare CMB, Rees M, Sainsburg MJ. Differentiation of two genetically specific types of depression by the response to antidepressants. Lancet 1962; *ii*: 1340-3.

29 Paykell ES. Depressive typologies and response to amitriptyline. Br J Psychiatry 1972; *120*: 147-56.

30 Pichot P, Lacassin J, Dreyfus JF. Essai de prédiction des indications de la nomifensine à partir du profil symptomatique pré-thérapeutique. Nouv Presse Méd 1978; *7*: 2313-6.

31 Prusoff BA, Paykel ES. Typological prediction of response to amitryptiline: a replication study. Pharmacopsychiatry 1977; *12*: 153-9.

32 Raskin A. The prediction of antidepressant drug effects : review and critique. In: Efron DH, Cole JO, Levine J et al, ed. Psychopharmacology: a review of progress. 1957-1967. Public Health Service Publication 1968; *n° 1836*: 757-65.

33 Raskin A, Schulterbrandt JG, Reating N, Chase C, McKean JJ. Differential response to chlorpromazine, imipramine and placebo. A study of subgroups of hospitalized patients. Arch Gen Psychiatry 1970; *23*: 164-73.

34 Raskin A, Boothe H, Schulterbrandt JG, Reating N, Odle D. A model for use in depressed patients. J Nerv Dis 1973; *156*: 130-42.

35 Raskin A, Schulterbrandt JG, Reating N, Crook TH, Odle D. Depression subtypes and response to phenelzine, diazepam and a placebo. Arch Gen Psychiatry 1974; *30*: 66-75.

36 Raskin A. Age-sex differences in response to antidepressant drugs. J Nerv Ment Dis 1974; *159*: 120-30.

37 Rasking A, Crook TH. Antidepressants in black and white patients. Arch Gen Psychiatry 1975; *32*: 643-9.

38 Rickels K, Gordon PE, Weise CC, Bazillian SE, Feldman HS, Wilson DA. Amitriptyline and trimipramine in neurotic depressed outpatients: a collaborative study. Amer J Psychiatry, 1970; *127*: 208-18.

39 Schildkraut JJ. Norepinephrine metabolites as biochemical criteria for classifying depressive disorders and predicting responses to treatment: preliminary findings. Amer J Psychiatry 1973; *130*: 695-9.

40 Schneider B. The role of hypothesis testing in clinical trials. Methods Information Medicine 1981; *20*: 65-6.

41 Schneider B. Analysis of clinical trial outcomes: alternative approaches to subgroup analysis. Controlled Clinical Trials 1989; *10*: 176S-86S.

42 Simes RJ. An improved Bonferroni procedure for multiple tests of significance. Biometrika 1986; *73*: 751-4.

43 Simon R. Patient subsets and variation in therapeutic efficacy. Br J Clin Pharmac 1982; *14*: 473-82.

44 Spriet A, Beiler D, Dechorgnat J, Chigot CD, Rossner M, Simon P. Méthodologie d'une étude cooperative des prédicteurs de réponse dans des syndromes dépressifs ambulatoires traités par la nomifensine. Nouv Presse Méd 1978; *7*: 2317-22.

45 Van Praag HM. Significance of biochemical parameters in the diagnosis, treatment and prevention of depressive disorders. Biological Psychiatry 1977; *12*: 101-31.

46 Weintraub M, Taves DR, Hasday JD, Mushlin AL, Lockwood DH. Determinants of response to anorexiants. Clin Pharmacol Ther 1981; *30*: 528-33.

47 Young MA, Foog LF. Predicting response to treatment: differentiating active factor and non-specific effects. Statistics in Medicine 1990; *9*: 253-61.

18 - "Pragmatic trials"
Decision methods

SUMMARY

The "pragmatic" trial is a global approach which incorporates considerations suited to this option on the selection of subjects and the methods of evaluation and which contrasts with the "explanatory" attitude of classical trials. Other methods with "known horizon" assume the total number of subjects who will receive a new treatment is known. Prior data can be incorporated into the strategy according to Bayes' method.

Decision methods make it possible to choose one of the treatments compared. They assume that it is possible to estimate the treatments based on the overall advantages and disadvantages and that an adequate number of cases are assembled to ensure a low probability that the treatment chosen is not "too much" less effective.

Decision methods do not permit a situation where no conclusion is made, nor to conclude on the equivalence of treatments.

In addition to traditional statistical analysis procedures (test of significance and the confidence interval), there are also other methods which serve as a guide in *choosing* between two or more treatments, based on data observations. These methods are referred to as *decisional* although this term is ambiguous since it can also be used in reference to traditional tests. The term *selection methods* may also be used.

1. PRINCIPLE

These methods imply the following:

• that a choice will be made after *quantitatively weighing* the advantages and disadvantages of the treatments,

• that no null hypothesis is formulated (no difference between the treatments or non-decision) but that the choice of a treatment (and rejection of the other or others) is based on results which suggest *that it is not less effective than the others by more than a pre-determined minimum difference and with a pre-determined probability or risk* (11, 12).

• that a choice will be made, even if there is no real difference between the treatments.

This implies:

• that if the *real* difference is less than the minimum difference chosen, we accept the risk of choosing the less effective treatment, with a probability higher than the chosen threshold,

• that if there is no difference, we must accept a decision based on chance alone since some choice has to be made anyway.

1.1. Advantages of these methods:

• there is no alternative but to make a choice, which *coincides with the reality* of medical prescribing,

• it is possible to make a *global* estimation of the treatments, based on their overall advantages and disadvantages,

• a conclusion can be reached with *fewer subjects* than with standard statistical analysis.

1.2. Disadvantages:

• a relatively arbitrary weight has to be assigned to the advantages and disadvantages of the treatments. Choosing different weights could in some cases lead to a different conclusion. This means that those in favor of the rejected treatment will probably find the decision unconvincing, leading to dispute or controversy (10),

• selection methods disregard negligible differences that should lead to a non-decision (15), at least while awaiting other results, or other advantages arising from the wide-scale or long-term use of a new treatment,

• a conclusion that the treatment selected is more effective than the other treatments compared cannot be made: the only possible conclusion is that it is not less effective.

2. PRINCIPAL METHODS

The main decision methods are shown in table I.

These methods seek to assemble a *sufficient number of cases* so that the treatment chosen (wrongly) is only less effective with a maximum probability decided upon in advance.

Table I The main decision methods

Authors	Number of treatments	Types of variables	References	Criterion of decision and procedure	
Schwartz, Flamant, Lellouch (pragmatic trial)	2	Gaussian distribution, Dichotomous response	(11, 12)	• Maximum probability of a wrong choice* if the true difference is equal to a minimum difference Δ • Possibility of an asymmetric choice with a "handicap" for one of the treatments owing to a disadvantage known independently of the trial.	2 procedures: • calculation of the number of subjects required, • sequential method
Hoel, Sobel, Weiss	2	Dichotomous response	(10, 13)	• Probability of correct selection • Possibility of an asymmetrical formulation	2 procedures: • two-step method: attribution by pairs, then "play the winner" method to minimize the number of subjects receiving the "less effective" method • sequential method
Bechhofer	= 2 ≥ 2	Gaussian distribution	(2, 3)	Minimum acceptable probability of correct classification	2 procedures: • calculation of the number of subjects required • sequential method
Sobel and Huyett	> 2	Dichotomous response	(13)	Correct probability of selection : maximum acceptable probability that the treatment chosen is less effective than the other treatments within a margin of Δ	Calculation of the number of subjects necessary
Taylor and David	> 2	Dichotomous response	(14)	Idem, and in addition, adaptive* allocation of treatments to minimize the number of subjects receiving the less effective treatment	
Berry and Pearson	2	Dichotomous response	(4)	Prior information available (probability of success).	• First step is comparative • Second step a treatment is selected (optimization of the number of success up to a "horizon".

* Adaptive methods of allocation of treatment achieve a variable distribution of patients (by treatment) during the trial depending on the proportion of success or failures of each treatment (10).

3. PRAGMATIC TRIAL (11, 12)

This original view on clinical trials differs from other methods presented in table I by a more global approach (table II).

Table II
The "pragmatic" and "explanatory" methods (11, 12)

	Pragmatic	Explanatory
Objective	To select one of the treatments	To answer a scientific question
Selection	Natural Broad	Homogeneous Reproducible
Prescription	Freely-adjusted Non-blind	Standardized Blind
Criterion	Comprehensive summary (weighting)	Evaluation of the effect (metrological qualities)
Sample size	Adequate to make choosing the " too much" less effective treatment a rare event.	Adequate so that if the difference is Δ, the test $(1 - \beta)$ is significant $(p \leq \alpha)$
Analysis	$\mathcal{P}$ (incorrect selection) $\leq \gamma$	Hypothesis-testing (Δ, α, β) and the confidence interval
Possible conclusions	One possible conclusion choice of A > B: it probably is not "too much less effective". It may either be: - better, - equivalent, - or slightly worse.	Four possible conclusions: - a significant difference in favour of the better treatment, - non-significant difference and a confidence interval between $+\Delta$ and $-\Delta$: equivalence, no choice, - non-significant difference and a confidence interval that overlaps either $+\Delta$ or $-\Delta$: exclusion of a major difference in a direction opposite from the result, - non-significant difference and a confidence interval that overlap $+\Delta$ and $-\Delta$: no conclusion can be drawn.

The authors of this method advocate its use in trials designed for practical applications as opposed to *explanatory* trials which, according to their point of view, are conducted for the purpose of scientific research.

In this scheme, priority is given:

-with *pragmatic* trials, to the selection of patients representative of the population to be treated rather than homogeneity of the groups. Emphasis is also placed on normal conditions of treatment rather than standardization,

- with *explanatory trials*, priority is given to the selection of subjects favoring sensitivity in demonstrating differences (hence a homogeneous selection of cases) and to standardization of treatments.

Although this classification is interesting, it probably has little application in the field of the study of a new drug before *registration*, where the purpose is mainly to look for the advantages of the new treatment. In other practical situations, where the problem is to eliminate the "worse" or "not better" treatment, it could have interesting applications.

4. METHODS WITH "KNOWN HORIZON"

Other procedures assume that the total number of subjects who will receive a new treatment - before another new therapy makes it obsolete - can be pre-determined.

The problem is then to reduce to a minimum the number of subjects, who receive the "inferior" tretament by optimizing the fraction of the total number of the patients who will be enrolled in the trial and subsequently to apply the decision (choice of the "not less effective" treatment), to the others (1, 5, 6, 7, 8). Although these methods are of theoretical interest, in practice they do not seem very compatible with what we currently know about the effective "lifespan" of a particular treatment.

In addition, it is possible in a *Bayesian* analysis to take into account prior information on the percentage of success of one or both of two treatments without knowing which one is better (4, 9).

References

1   Anscombe FJ. Sequential medical trials. J Amer Statist Assoc 1963; *58*: 365-83.

2   Bechhofer RE, Dunett CW, Sobel M. A two-sample multiple decision procedure for ranking means of normal populations with a common unknown variance. Biometrika 1954; *41*: 170-6.

3   Bechhofer RE. A sequential multiple-decision procedure for selecting the best one of several normal populations with unknown variance and its use with various experimental designs. Biometrics 1958; *14*: 408-29.

4   Berry DA, Pearson LM. Optimal designs for clinical trials with dichotomous responses. Statistics in Medicine 1985; *4*: 497-508.

5   Canner PL. Selecting one of two treatments when the responses are dichotomous. J Amer Statist Assoc 1970; *65*: 293-306.

6   Colton T. A model for selecting one of two medical treatments. J Amer Statist Assoc 1963; *58*: 388-400.

7   Cornfield J, Halperin M, Greenhouse SW. An adaptive procedure for sequential clinical trials. J Amer Statist Assoc 1969; *64*: 759-70.

8   Donner A. The use of auxiliary information in the design of a clinical trial. Biometrics 1977; *33*: 305-14.

9   Feinstein AR. Clinical biostatistics XXXIX. The haze of Bayes, the aerial balances of decision analysis and the computerized Ouija board. Clin Pharmacol Ther 1977; *21*: 482-96.

10 Hoel DG, Sobel M, Weiss GH. A survey of adaptive sampling in clinical trials. In: Elashoff R M, ed: Perspectives in Biometry; *Vol 1*: Academic Press, 1975.

11 Schwartz D, Lellouch J. Explanatory and pragmatic attitudes in therapeutic trials. J Chron Dis 1967; *20*: 637-48.

12 Schwartz D, Flamant R, Lellouch J. L'essai thérapeutique chez l'homme. Flammarion, 1970.

13 Sobel M, Huyett M. Selecting the best of several binomial populations. Bell System Tech J 1957; *36*: 537-76.

14 Taylor TJ, David HA. A multistage procedure for the selection of the best of several populations. J Amer Statist Assoc 1962; *57*: 785-96.

15 Tukey JW. Conclusions vs decisions. Technometrics 1960; *2*: 423-33.

19 - Safety data

SUMMARY

• *The collection of data on drug safety must be made differently for serious accidents (which require detailed information) and for minor events which are systematically sought. Laboratory data on drug safety must be interpreted according to the methods of assay and the normal values used.*

• *Assessment of the causal relationship may be facilitated by systematic algorithms.*

• *Analysis of data on safety must consider the comparisons of frequency, changes in frequency, the probability of observing at least one case for a given sample size, and the timing of onset.*

During a clinical trial, the collection of adverse events is of major importance to assess the efficacy/safety ratio, although most often this is not the principal criterion of the study (pool of data collected during several trials is necessary). We shall not discuss administrative and regulatory procedures (emergency alert system, reporting, centralization, circulation) nor coding of data (necessary for computer processing of open questions), but rather the methodological aspects relating to the collection, interpretation and analysis of data on safety.

1. COLLECTION

Among adverse events, a distinction is made between minor events and major or serious ones. The latter have been defined in official texts (notably in the USA and in Europe).

For the european guidelines, "a serious adverse event means an adverse experience that is fatal, life-threatening, disabling or which results in in-patient hospitalization or prolongation of hospitalization. In addition, congenital anomaly and occurence of malignancy are always considered serious adverse events" (1).

All the steps and forms for:
- the verification of the recording of adverse events,
- the emergency-alert system, documentation, assessment of the causal relationship, and reporting of serious adverse events must be specified in written procedures which are not part of the methodology but rather are part of good practices (15).

1.1. Serious adverse events

Serious adverse events which occur during a clinical trial may be recorded in a standardized form, which generally is derived from the CIOMS form (Council of International Organization of Medical Sciences) or from the Food and Drug Administration (18). It is wise and practical to provide one such form per case report form. Thus, the investigator does not have to search through a study book (kept heaven knows where) or to ask the sponsor for it. His task thus is simplified.

1.2. Minor adverse events

Minor adverse events must always be recorded at each visit so that their chronology may easily be followed-up (regression, onset, worsening...). This can be done in several ways:

• either by open collection of such events, recording the effects which the subject complains about spontaneously, possibly after routine questioning of the patient using a standardized question such as "Have you experienced any discomfort with this medication?",

• or in the form of a closed questionnaire used to systematically question the patient about the development of an entire series of symptoms contained in a pre-determined list.

The first procedure has the disadvantage of not knowing the effects which the patient does not complain of spontaneously, the second has the drawback of suggesting symptoms to the patient and of increasing the incidence of adverse events, many of which are influenced or induced by a mechanism that is purely psychological ("nocebo" effect). [*]

However, in a comparative trial, it matters little that there is an exaggerated incidence of subjective complaints; what is important is not to favor such complaints with one treatment rather than with another. Moreover, although a closed questionnaire increases the incidence of adverse events mentioned in the list, it *decreases the frequency of events not contained in the list*.

A compromise may be found by first using an open questionnaire followed by a closed list in successive order.

It is important not to record only adverse *effects* (presumably due to treatment), but all abnormal *events* regardless of their presumable causal relationship, because the interpretation can change as data accumulate (for

[*] Some protocols specify the incorporation in a closed list of "unlikely" effects to identify persons easily influenced by suggestion.

220

example, cough and administration of angiotensin converting enzyme inhibitors). Nonetheless, it is difficult to know when to stop so as not to collect an overabundance of pointless and unusable information (20).

In addition, some pre-existing symptoms of a disorder may be erroneously interpreted as adverse events due to treatment if they have not been screened for routinely at the start of the trial. Thus, it is desirable to also fill out the list of "side-effects" *prior to treatment* !

In all cases, the *severity and outcome* of any adverse event must be recorded as well as the decision taken (change in dosage or discontinuation of treatment).

1.3. Laboratory test safety

It should be kept in mind that an abnormal laboratory test value may be a minor or a major adverse event.

Laboratory tests of safety are collected at least once prior to treatment (results of such tests are often part of eligibility criteria) and in the final evaluation. An adequate place will of course be provided in the case report forms for recording laboratory safety tests specified in the protocol. Most commonly this involves one standard sheet per visit. Methods of assays and limits considered as normal for values by the laboratory performing the tests are collected independently for all corresponding cases (generally by center). In case of a minor abnormal laboratory test value, it is wise to ask the investigator his opinion on the clinical relevance of the result. This can be done by providing a box to be checked off as "yes", provided with each laboratory test result requested.

2. CAUSAL RELATIONSHIP

Several methods have been proposed to assess in a reproducible manner the degree of certainty of the causal relationship of the study medication and the adverse event. No method is perfectly satisfactory: the best method is the one to which one is accustomed .

2.1. The Karch and Lasagna method (10)

This method is based on a decision-tree consisting of five criteria (timing, previously-known event, other possible cause, outcome following termination of treatment and rechallenge). It results in six ratings: definite relation, probable, possible, conditional, doubtful, negative. It is used by the Food and Drug Administration but is not compulsory in the USA.

2.2. The Kramer et al. method (8, 11)

This method uses a very complete decision-tree, making it possible to take into consideration many more varied and precise shades of meaning than YES or NO answers.

Nevertheless, this method is relatively complicated and assumes that a procedure be followed through several very complete diagrams. Thus, it is very rarely used in routine practice.

2.3. The French method (4, 5)

This method is based on the combination:

- of chronological criteria:
• time of onset of the event: very suggestive, compatible, or incompatible,
• rechallenge with the study drug (positive with recurrence of the event, not done, not evaluable or negative, i.e. no recurrence of the event),
• outcome upon cessation of treatment with the drug: highly suggestive (regression coinciding with termination), inconclusive, or unknown.

- criteria based on clinical manifestations:
• clinical or laboratory manifestations suggesting the role of the suspect medication, reliable specific investigations (positive, not available, or negative test result),
• no other explanation (after appropriate assessment) or possible (not detected or present).

All these criteria lead to assignment of a chronological score (C1 to C3) and of a score of symptoms (S1 to S3) which combine in the overall score for assessment of an "intrinsic causal relationship" (I1 to I4). It is compulsory to use this method in France for post-marketing data.

2.4. The Bayes method (3, 6, 7, 12)

It enables estimation of the likelihood of the causal relationship by integrating the following items:

- the relationship for the incidences of the adverse event with and without the suspect drug,
- the likelihood ratios of features collected on the case (symptoms, chronology, rechallenge).

This prior information is either drawn from previous experience or from epidemiological studies, or is the subject of arbitrary assumptions (based on known facts concerning drugs in the same therapeutic class). In this case, it is wise to test several hypotheses, hoping that the conclusion is "robust" (little sensitivity to the assumptions made). This method, used especially in drug safety monitoring to assess the causal relationship of known events, offers little opportunity in the context of a clinical trial with a new drug since the basic information is still too incomplete.

3. STATISTICAL QUESTIONS

Several questions may be asked (16, 17):

3.1. Frequency

The frequency of an adverse effect is theoretically obtained simply by relating the number of cases observed to the number of subjects exposed. Nonetheless, detection of cases may not be comprehensive, and artifacts (cases not due to the product) can be included erroneously. Ideally, a frequency should be assessed by giving its confidence interval, for example a 95% confidence interval, which of course becomes that much narrower as there is a large number of subjects.

3.2. Increased frequency

An event may be considered as being rare at the start of development of a product, and then prove to be more frequent. It then is appropriate to monitor the development of new cases in all of the ongoing trials, possibly by computerized methods (19).

3.3. Sample size "to observe one case"

To have a reasonable chance (for example 95%) of observing at least one instance of a rare adverse event, it is possible to calculate the necessary number of subjects exposed. If the true frequency is 1/N, the probability of observing at least one case will be 95% if the number of subjects exposed is equal to 3N. If the number of cases observed is greater than 1, the sample size necessary is given in table I.

Table I
Detection of rare events : number of subjects necessary.

Number of cases of the adverse event	Probability of detection		
	0.90	0.95	0.99
≥ 1	2.3 N	3.0 N	4.6 N
≥ 2	3.9 N	4.8 N	6.6 N
≥ 3	5.3 N	6.3 N	8.4 N
≥ 4	6.7 N	7.8 N	10.1 N
≥ 5	8.0 N	9.2 N	11.6 N

If the frequency of the effect is 1 for N subjects exposed, the table provides the coefficient by which N must be multiplied to observe a given number of cases (lines) with a given probability (columns).

3.4. Maximum frequency possible

If no serious adverse event has been observed with a sample size of N subjects, it is possible to calculate the maximum frequency compatible with a 95% confidence interval, if it is approximately equal to 3/N (95% confidence interval between 0 and 3/N). More exactly, f max = $1 - \sqrt[N]{0.05}$ (table II).

Table II
Upper limit of confidence

No event was observed in N cases : upper limit of confidence (ULC) at P%	
P	**ULC**
99%	$\dfrac{4.6}{N}$
95%	$\dfrac{3}{N}$
90%	$\dfrac{2.3}{N}$

3.5. Comparison of frequencies of adverse events

Comparison of frequencies is possible in controlled trials only for frequent effects. Generally, the power of tests involving adverse events is poor in comparison to the power of comparison for efficacy, and a "non-significant" difference doesn't mean much if the result is not accompanied by the confidence interval of the difference. Sometimes, acceptable combinations of adverse events may be made (by organ system or by symptom) to increase the power of the analysis. Common analysis of several trials for this type of test is possible only if the treatments compared are the same and the protocols are compatible.

3.6. "Life-table" (time-to-event analysis) (2, 9, 13, 14)

The frequency of an adverse event does not provide sufficient information to understand it well and to recommend a monitoring strategy. It is also necessary to know the timing of its onset. To assess both the frequency and the time of onset, a "life-table" (time-to-event analysis) may be constructed by calculating stepwise the probability of onset of an adverse event for increasing durations of treatment. Thus, adverse events may occur with three different patterns:
- adverse events developing especially at the beginning of treatment and rarely afterward (the cumulative probability curve increases then stabilizes),
- effects whose frequency is independent of the duration of treatment (the curve increases progressively),
- adverse events developing only after a prolonged period of treatment (figure 1)

Figure 1
Adverse events
life-table method
(13,14)

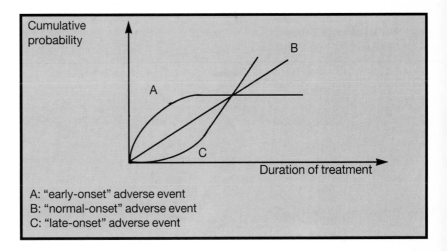

Cumulative probability

B

A

C

Duration of treatment

A: "early-onset" adverse event
B: "normal-onset" adverse event
C: "late-onset" adverse event

If the adverse event may have major consequences: in the first case, intensive monitoring is recommended at the beginning of treatment and constant monitoring in the second case. In the latter case, it may be necessary to recommend treatment for short periods only.

4. CONCLUSIONS

Knowledge concerning the tolerability of a drug is primarily an evolving process: very frequent effects will be detected during phase I trials and they are decisive factors in determining whether development of the drug should continue. Then each study provides a certain amount of information. In the clinical file for drug registration it is the combined analysis of tolerability of all trials (table III) which enables correct evaluation of frequencies and finally comparing them with that of other treatments. Post-marketing drug surveillance alone makes possible the detection of rare events (from a frequency less than 1 in a thousand) in the very large sample of patients exposed to such events. These methods differ from those of clinical trials in which more commonly fewer patients are involved.

Table III
Pooled analysis of tolerability.
Adverse events (A.E.) in all trials
within a clinical file

Adverse events
• Patients with no adverse events (number as a %)
• Tabulation by organ or by system
- All A.E.
- Minor A.E.
- Serious A.E.
• Tabulation of frequent A.E.
• Comparison treatment-control (tests, confidence intervals)
• Frequency by dose:
- titration studies
- dose-response studies
• Frequency by duration of treatments: life-tables
• Description of each serious event with: clinical manifestations, dose, duration, outcome
Laboratory tests
• Out of range values (number and %)
• Outcome, trends (curves, tests, "before-after")
• Description of serious abnormalities
Other data of tolerability
• Vital signs
• Special tests (ophthalmological, ECG, etc...)

References

1 Anonymous. Bonnes pratiques cliniques pour les essais de médicaments dans la Communauté Européenne. 4ème colloque DPhM. INSERM. L'Europe du médicament: réalités et ambitions. INSERM 1990; *213*: 433-74.

2 Abt K, Cockburn ITR, Guelich A, Krupp P. Evaluation of adverse reactions by means of the life-table method. Drug Information Journal 1989; *23*: 143-9.

3 Auriche M. Approche bayésienne de l'imputabilité des phénomènes indésirables aux médicaments. Thérapie 1985; *40*: 301-6.

4 Bégaud B, Evreux JC, Jouglard J, Lagier G. Imputabilité des effets inattendus ou toxiques des médicaments. Actualisation de la méthode utilisée en France. Thérapie 1985; *40*: 111-4.

5 Bégaud B, Evreux JC, Jouglard J, Lagier G. Unexpected or toxic drug reaction assessment (imputation). Actualization of the method used in France. Thérapie 1985; *40*: 115-22.

6 Hutchinson TA, David AP, Spiegelhalter DJ, Cowell RG, Roden S. Computerized aids for probabilistic assessment of drug safety. I: A spreadsheet program. Drug Information Journal 1991; *25*: 29-39.

7 Hutchinson TA, David AP, Spiegelhalter DJ, Cowell RG, Roden S. Computerized aids for probabilistic assessment of drug safety. II: An expert system. Drug Information Journal 1991; *25*: 41-8.

8 Hutchinson TA, Leventhal JM, Kramer MS, Karch FE, Lipman AG, Feinstein AR. An algorithm for the operational assessment of adverse drug reactions. II: Demonstration of reproducibility and validity. J Amer Med Assoc 1979; *242*: 633-8.

9 Idanpaan-Heikkila J. A review of safety information obtained from phases I-II and phase III. Clinical investigations of sixteen selected drugs. Washington: US Government Printing Office. Food and Drug Administration, 1983.

10 Karch FE, Lasagna L. Toward the operational identification of adverse drug reactions. Clin Pharmacol Ther 1977; *21*: 247-54.

11 Kramer MS, Leventhal JM, Hutchinson TA, Feinstein AR. An algorithm for the operational assessment of adverse drug reactions. I. Background, description and instructions for use. JAMA 1979; *242*: 632-6.

12 Lane DA, Kramer MS, Hutchinson TA, Jones JK, Naranjo C. The causality assessment of adverse drug reactions using a Bayesian approach. Pharmaceut Med 1987; 2: 265-83.

13 O'Neill RT. Statistical analyses of adverse events, data from clinical trials, special emphasis on serious events. Drug Information Journal, 1987; 21: 9-20.

14 O'Neill RT. Assessment of safety. In: Karl E. Peace. Biopharmaceutical statistics for drug development. New York: Marcel Dekker, 1988.

15 Spriet A, Dupin-Spriet T. a) Bonne pratique des essais cliniques des médicaments. Bâle: Karger 1990. b) Good practice of clinical drug trials. Basel: Karger, 1992.

16 Spriet-Pourra C, Spriet A, Soubrié C, Simon P. Les méthodes d'étude des effets indésirables des médicaments. I: Recueil des données et types d'études. Thérapie 1981; 36: 609-18.

17 Spriet-Pourra C, Spriet A, Soubrié C, Simon P. Les méthodes d'étude des effets indésirables des médicaments. II: Questions relatives aux fréquences. Thérapie 1982; 37: 13-22

18 Stephens MDB. The detection of new adverse drug reactions. New York: Stockton Press, 1988.

19 Tangrea JA, Adrianza ME, McAdams M. A method for the detection and management of adverse events in clinical trials. Drug Information Journal 1991; 25: 63-80.

20 Weintraub M. Recording events in clinical trials. Br Med J 1978; 1: 581.

20 - Sample size

SUMMARY

The sample size determines the probability of detecting a difference between the treatments compared in a controlled trial. The number of subjects must be large:

• to demonstrate a small difference;

• if there will be a marked variability in the results;

• if the acceptable probability of a false positive result will be low (difference due to chance alone);

• if the level of certainty required (1 - ß) for the detection of a given difference will be high (i.e. close to certainty).

Formulas for calculating sample size necessarily use arbitrary values for each of these factors and provide only an approximation of the number of subjects required.

Other factors also intervene, notably the rate of attrition of subjects during a trial, the experimental design, unequal randomization, one or two-tailed tests, and intermediate analyses.

Before concluding that the treatments compared do not differ noticeably and that they are equivalent within a range of negligible difference, checks must be made to ensure that the number of subjects was in fact sufficient to detect a given true difference.

One of the first questions to be considered when undertaking a controlled trial is the number of subjects required. However, it is often impossible to give a valid answer to this question until the results of the trial are known! The question might well be divided into subquestions as follows:

• How much does the number of subjects influence the results ?

• At what point is it possible to estimate (at least approximately) the number of subjects required if the intended trial is to provide a valid result?

• When the trial is completed, can one draw an *a posteriori* conclusion that the number of subjects is large enough to draw conclusions?

1. FACTORS DETERMINING THE NUMBER OF SUBJECTS

The number of subjects required for a comparative trial depends on the following factors:

• The degree of sensitivity aimed at in the comparison. The smaller the difference one wishes to demonstrate, the more subjects one needs. When comparing treatments that *barely* differ from each other, a much larger number of subjects is required than when attempting to demonstrate a marked difference.

In some cases, one might wish to demonstrate a very small difference since any therapeutic progress, however small, should not be overlooked. For practical purposes, a *realistic compromise* has to be found. This means arbitrarily setting a limit between the difference one accepts to ignore and the difference one wishes to demonstrate with a reasonable degree of certainty.

• On the *variability* (or "variance") *of the results*. If the results differ very little from one patient to another, far fewer subjects will be required than when the responses to treatment vary widely. For a given sensitivity of the comparison, the required number of subjects may therefore be lowered by reducing the variability using all possible means:

- by recruiting groups which are homogeneous in terms of those characteristics likely to affect the results;

- by interpreting the results on the basis of sensitive, precise and reproducible criteria;

- by standardizing as much as possible the conditions under which the treatments studied are administered.

Even after taking all these precautions, there is always a degree of variability in the results that cannot be eliminated. The extent and importance of this variability can only be determined after all the data have been collected. Ideally, the exact variance should have been available at the start of the trial to allow calculation of the number of subjects required. In this less than ideal world, the only alternative is to *predict* the approximate variability of the results:

- either based on a previous trial carried out under circumstances as comparable as possible to those of the intended trial. Previous trial data may even be used to plot power curves which indicate the probability of detecting a given difference (10, 31);

Table I   Main methods for calculating sample size

Type of variables Statistical test	Method for calculating sample size	References	Remarks
Binary (dichotomous) 2 samples χ^2	Normal approximation Arc-sine approximation Taking into account correction for continuity	(34) (7, 16) (35, 44)	Number of subjects underestimated for small samples (7)
Exact probability	Exact test: table	(16, 20)	
Qualitative Contingency table with one row and c columns: χ^2		(27)	
Comparison of 2 means Gaussian variables	Algorithm Normal approximation t test algorithm (successive approximations) Estimation of variance on a previous sample - algorithm - tables - graph	(34) (39) (21) (14) (9) (2)	
Paired or within-patient design **Paired t test**		(34)	The algorithm requires a value for the correlation coefficient between the two successive measurements in the same subject. In fact, in a cross-over trial, for analysis of results, ANOVA is used which takes into account the "period effect".
Comparison of several means		(15)	
Analysis of variance	Graphs Tables	(8,14,32) (3, 23, 24, 25, 26)	Requires a "non-centrality parameter" taking into account the variance of the means; allows determination of ß from the value of N. Determination of N as a function of the difference between the maximum and minimum means for: - parallel groups - randomized blocks
Comparison of two survival curves		(18, 31, 36, 40, 42, 46)	Δ = ratio of mean survival times. The tables make it possible to determine the number of subjects and the duration of the trial.

- or whenever possible, based on a pilot study which gives an approximate idea of the variance of the results, and provides a means of testing the "feasibility" of the trial. However, such pilot studies cause delays in starting the actual trial.

If the treatments are to be compared over a long period of time - sometimes several years - undertaking a proper pilot study would be too lengthy a process. The only solution, for lack of a better substitute, is therefore either to extrapolate the results of shorter treatment periods, or to undertake a retrospective analysis of patients who have been studied for a sufficient length of time, but for whom different treatments were prescribed...

• On the level of significance α of the statistical comparison which is considered meaningful. When we are seeking a low probability that the difference observed can be attributed to random fluctuations alone, then the number of subjects must be proportionately higher. Here again, the level should ideally be as low as possible, but compromises are necessary.

• *On the degree of probability of not missing a true difference.* Once again, the smaller the number of subjects, the greater the risk of error β one must be prepared to accept.

When deciding on the number of participants, several additional factors have to be taken into consideration:

• unequal randomization which results in a loss of power, actually relatively low if the imbalance is not too marked (17) (table II);

Table II
Unequal randomization

Number of subjects necessary to obtain power equal to that of equal numbers of subjects	
Proportion in the two groups	Increase in total number of subjects
$\frac{1}{2} + \frac{1}{2}$	0
$\frac{2}{3} + \frac{1}{3}$	+12,5%
$\frac{3}{4} + \frac{1}{4}$	+33%
$\frac{4}{5} + \frac{1}{5}$	+56%
$\frac{5}{6} + \frac{1}{6}$	+80%
$\frac{6}{7} + \frac{1}{7}$	+100%

• the experimental design: in particular, in a crossover trial, the same patients are used twice;

• attrition resulting from subjects lost to follow-up for whom information is lost which must be compensated for (if p is the proportion of subjects lost to follow-up, the number of subjects must be increased by a factor of 1/1-p),

• failure to comply with the treatments, which lowers their efficacy, increases the variability and decreases any differences which might exist between the groups (39),

• the statistical method chosen. If it is possible to choose between several tests, the most *powerful* method requires smaller numbers of subjects,

• Possible choice of a one-tailed test, provided that the hypothesis tested allows this to be done (chapter 2), which requires a smaller number of subjects,

• some methods of intermediate analysis which result, although they compensate fo α level inflation, in a loss of power of the final test, to be compensated for (chapter 16).

Finally, although a larger number of subjects may make it possible to demonstrate a small difference in efficacy between the treatments, unfortunately, it also renders it susceptible to bias: groups that are not comparable, assessment criteria that favor or disfavor one of the treatments compared, treatments administered under conditions which give an advantage to one treatment or another. In case of *bias*, the larger the number of subjects, the more erroneous the result!

2. FORMULAS FOR CALCULATING THE NUMBER OF SUBJECTS

Theoretically, for a given *statistical method chosen to analyze the results*, one can calculate the number of subjects required to demonstrate a given difference by taking the above-mentioned factors into account (28).

If we keep in mind the arbitrary nature of the values or the entirely relative accuracy of an estimation of variables or constants included in the formulas, the result must never be considered as anything more than an *approximate idea* of the required number of subjects.

This sometimes makes it obvious that the hypotheses tested are unrealistic, in that the number of subjects required far exceeds the available means, or that the therapeutic improvement desired is out of all proportion to the effort involved.

There are three logical conclusions in this situation:

• either that the trial should not be done;

• that a much greater effort will have to be made than had been anticipated, for example by planning a multicenter trial;

• or that we should restrict ourselves to testing less ambitious hypotheses.

In fact, we often actually use the opposite method of calculating the required number of subjects to the one mentioned above. That is to say we consider the number of subjects that can be recruited and we examine the values of α, β, and Δ that can be expected, which then enables us to decide if this particular trial is justified.

The calculation formulas themselves are far beyond the scope of this book. *Table I* shows the available methods and provides the interested reader with the necessary references for finding a simple algorithm, tables or graphs.

Among the most pertinent of the existing statistical methods, many have no simple corresponding techniques for calculating sample size, often because it is difficult to formulate a clear alternative hypothesis. Therefore, *in order to obtain an approximate idea* of the required number of subjects, we sometimes use a process which in fact corresponds to a simpler statistical test. Sometimes, simulations provide a better approach in complex cases (22).

3. SIMPLE METHOD FOR THE MOST FREQUENT CASES

3.1. Principle

Tables IIIa to IIIc make it possible by simple multiplication of 2 terms (C_1 and C_2) to obtain the approximate number of subjects necessary per group for a parallel group trial with two treatments for a qualitative criterion and for a normal variable, for a one or two-tailed test, and for an "equivalence" trial.

Approximate calculation of the number of cases :

$N = C_1 \times C_2$ per group
C_1 = depends on the difference that one wishes to detect
C_2 = depends on values chosen for α and β

Table IIIa can be used for the comparison of two means (test or equivalence) and allows calculation of sample size, from:
Δ = value chosen as the arbitrary limit between an "interesting" difference and a "negligible" difference.
σ : standard deviation: square root of the variance (mean of the squares of deviations from the population mean).
C_1 is obtained from $\frac{\Delta}{\sigma}$ and C_2 from α and β.

Table IIIb (comparison of two proportions, one- and two-tailed tests).
From P_0 (proportions of successes - assumed to be known - with the control therapy), and P_1 (expected proportion of success with the new therapy), coefficients are obtained and their difference is C_1. C_2 is obtained from α and β.

Table IIIc (equivalence trial for two proportions around P_0).
C_1 is obtained directly from P_1 and C_2 from Δ (acceptable limit of equivalence) for 90% or 95% confidence intervals.

3.2. Examples of calculation of sample size

• <u>Example 1:</u> How many subjects are needed in a trial on antihypertensive drugs, to demonstrate a difference of 5 mm Hg between two treatments with a standard deviation of 10 mm Hg by a two-tailed test with $\alpha = 0.05$ and $\beta = 0.10$?

Table III a:

Table for approximate sample sizes: comparison of two means

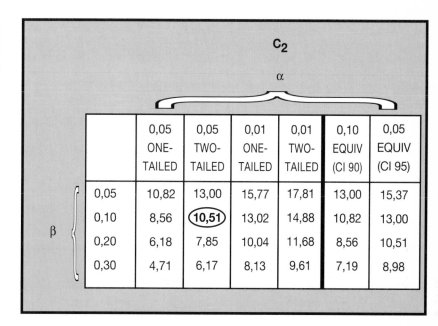

$\frac{\Delta}{\sigma}$	C_1
0.05	800.00
0.10	200.00
0.15	88.89
0.20	50.00
0.25	32.00
0.30	22.22
0.35	16.33
0.40	12.50
0.45	9.88
→ 0.50	8.00 ←
0.55	6.61
0.60	5.56
0.65	4.73
0.70	4.08
0.75	3.56
0.80	3.13
0.85	2.77
0.90	2.47
0.95	2.22
1.00	2.00
1.05	1.81
1.10	1.65
1.15	1.51
1.20	1.39
1.25	1.28
1.30	1.18
1.35	1.10
1.40	1.02
1.45	0.95
1.50	0.89
1.55	0.83
1.60	0.78
1.65	0.73
1.70	0.69
1.75	0.65
1.80	0.62
1.85	0.58
1.90	0.55
1.95	0.53
2.00	0.50

The C_2 table:

β	0,05 ONE-TAILED	0,05 TWO-TAILED	0,01 ONE-TAILED	0,01 TWO-TAILED	0,10 EQUIV (CI 90)	0,05 EQUIV (CI 95)
0,05	10,82	13,00	15,77	17,81	13,00	15,37
0,10	8,56	(10,51)	13,02	14,88	10,82	13,00
0,20	6,18	7,85	10,04	11,68	8,56	10,51
0,30	4,71	6,17	8,13	9,61	7,19	8,98

Δ = minimum difference to be detected with power 1- ß

σ = standard deviation

$N = C_1 \times C_2$

Example 1 (cont'd)

$\Delta = 5 \qquad \sigma = 10$

$$\frac{\Delta}{\sigma} = \frac{5}{10} = 0.5 \Rightarrow C_1$$

C_1 (left table) $\doteq$ 8 (arrows)

C_2 = 10.51 (circled)

N = 8 x 10.51 = 84 per group approximately

In order to demonstrate equivalence (probability ß that the 90% or 95% confidence interval lies entirely between +Δ and -Δ) the C_2 coefficients are found in the last two columns.

Table III b:
Table for approximate
sample sizes.
Comparison of two proportions
(significance test)

Example:
Frequency of the event with
control therapy = 20%
Expected gain = 10%

P_0, P_1	C_0	P_0, P_1	C_0
0	3142	51	1551
1	2941	52	1531
2	2858	53	1511
3	2793	54	1491
4	2739	55	1471
5	2691	56	1451
6	2647	57	1430
7	2606	58	1410
8	2568	59	1390
P1 9	2532	60	1369
►10	2498 ◄	61	1349
11	2465	62	1328
12	2434	63	1308
13	2404	64	1287
14	2375	65	1266
15	2346	66	1245
16	2319	67	1224
17	2292	68	1203
18	2265	69	1181
P0 19	2240	70	1159
►20	2214 ◄	71	1137
21	2190	72	1115
22	2165	73	1093
23	2141	74	1070
24	2118	75	1047
25	2094	76	1024
26	2071	77	1000
27	2049	78	976
28	2026	79	952
29	2004	80	927
30	1982	81	902
31	1961	82	876
32	1939	83	850
33	1918	84	823
34	1897	85	795
35	1875	86	767
36	1855	87	738
37	1834	88	707
38	1813	89	676
39	1793	90	644
40	1772	91	609
41	1752	92	574
42	1731	93	536
43	1711	94	495
44	1691	95	451
45	1671	96	403
46	1651	97	348
47	1631	98	284
48	1611	99	200
49	1591	100	000
50	1571		

• This page:
C_0 coefficients correspond to proportions P_0 (frequency of the event with the control therapy) and P_1 (frequency with the test treatment). Calculate the difference d between these two coefficients C_0.

• Next page:
For different values of d (10 to 1400) corresponding C_1 coefficient

• The sample size is obtained :
by multiplying C_1 by C_2 given by the table (below) for different values of α and ß.

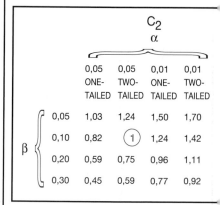

		0,05 ONE-TAILED	0,05 TWO-TAILED	0,01 ONE-TAILED	0,01 TWO-TAILED
ß	0,05	1,03	1,24	1,50	1,70
	0,10	0,82	(1)	1,24	1,42
	0,20	0,59	0,75	0,96	1,11
	0,30	0,45	0,59	0,77	0,92

Example 2:
Which sample size is needed for a survival trial if the expected rate of death is 20%, that the new treatment is hoped to reduce to 10% with a two-tailed test, $\alpha = 0.05$ and ß = 0.10?

Corresponding values for C_0 are 2498 and 2214 (arrows). Their difference is d = 284. Corresponding value for C_1 is 261 (arrows).
For a test wih $\alpha = 0.05$ and ß = 0.10, C_2 coefficient is 1 (circled). The sample size <u>by group</u> is 261 x 1 = <u>261</u>

Table III b (cont'd)

d	C1	d	C1	d	C1	d	C1	d	C1	d	C1	d	C1	d	C1
20	52540	74	3838	156	864	264	302	372	152	600	58	940	24	1960	5
21	47655	75	3736	158	842	266	297	374	150	605	57	950	23	1980	5
22	43421	76	3638	160	821	268	293	376	149	610	56	960	23	2000	5
23	39728	77	3545	162	801	270	288	378	147	615	56	970	22	2040	5
24	36486	78	3454	164	781	272	284	380	146	620	55	980	22	2080	5
25	33626	79	3367	166	763	274	280	382	144	625	54	990	21	2120	5
26	31089	80	3284	168	745	276	276	384	143	630	53	1000	21	2160	5
27	28828	81	3203	170	727	278	272	386	141	635	52	1020	20	2200	4
28	26806	82	3126	172	710	280	268	388	140	640	51	1040	19	2240	4
29	24989	83	3051	174	694	282	264	390	138	645	51	1060	19	2280	4
30	23351	84	2978	176	678	►284	261◄	392	137	650	50	1080	18	2320	4
31	21869	85	2909	178	663	286	257	394	135	655	49	1100	17	2360	4
32	20523	86	2842	180	649	288	253	396	134	660	48	1120	17	2400	4
33	19298	87	2777	182	634	290	250	398	133	665	48	1140	16	2440	4
34	18180	88	2714	184	621	292	246	400	131	670	47	1160	16	2480	3
35	17156	89	2653	186	607	294	243	405	128	675	46	1180	15	2520	3
36	16216	90	2595	188	595	296	240	410	125	680	45	1200	15	2560	3
37	15351	91	2538	190	582	298	237	415	122	685	45	1220	14	2600	3
38	14554	92	2483	192	570	300	234	420	119	690	44	1240	14	2640	3
39	13817	93	2430	194	558	302	230	425	116	695	44	1260	13	2680	3
40	13135	94	2378	196	547	304	227	430	114	700	43	1280	13	2720	3
41	12502	95	2329	198	536	306	224	435	111	705	42	1300	12	2760	3
42	11914	96	2280	200	525	308	222	440	109	710	42	1320	12	2800	3
43	11366	97	2234	202	515	310	219	445	106	715	41	1340	12	2840	3
44	10855	98	2188	204	505	312	216	450	104	720	41	1360	11	2880	3
45	10378	99	2144	206	495	314	213	455	102	725	40	1380	11	2920	2
46	9932	100	2102	208	486	316	210	460	99	730	39	1400	11	2960	2
47	9514	102	2020	210	477	318	208	465	97	735	39	1420	10	3000	2
48	9122	104	1943	212	468	320	205	470	95	740	38	1440	10	3040	2
49	8753	106	1870	214	459	322	203	475	93	745	38	1460	10	3080	2
50	8406	108	1802	216	450	324	200	480	91	750	37	1480	10	3120	2
51	8080	110	1737	218	442	326	198	485	89	755	37	1500	9	3160	2
52	7772	112	1675	220	434	328	195	490	88	760	36	1520	9	3200	2
53	7482	114	1617	222	426	330	193	495	86	765	36	1540	9	3240	2
54	7207	116	1562	224	419	332	191	500	84	770	35	1560	9	3280	2
55	6947	118	1509	226	411	334	188	505	82	775	35	1580	8	3320	2
56	6702	120	1459	228	404	336	186	510	81	780	35	1600	8	3360	2
57	6468	122	1412	230	397	338	184	515	79	785	34	1620	8	3400	2
58	6247	124	1367	232	390	340	182	520	78	790	34	1640	8	3440	2
59	6037	126	1324	234	384	342	180	525	76	795	33	1660	8	3480	2
60	5838	128	1283	236	377	344	178	530	75	800	33	1680	7	3520	2
61	5648	130	1244	238	371	346	176	535	73	810	32	1700	7	3560	2
62	5467	132	1206	240	365	348	174	540	72	820	31	1720	7	3600	2
63	5295	134	1170	242	359	350	172	545	71	830	31	1740	7	3640	2
64	5131	136	1136	244	353	352	170	550	69	840	30	1760	7	3680	2
65	4974	138	1104	246	347	354	168	555	68	850	29	1780	7	3720	2
66	4825	140	1072	248	342	356	166	560	67	860	28	1800	6	3760	1
67	4682	142	1042	250	336	358	164	565	66	870	28	1820	6		
68	4545	144	1014	252	331	360	162	570	65	880	27	1840	6		
69	4414	146	986	254	326	362	160	575	64	890	27	1860	6		
70	4289	148	959	256	321	364	159	580	62	900	26	1880	6		
71	4169	150	934	258	316	366	157	585	61	910	25	1900	6		
72	4054	152	910	260	311	368	155	590	60	920	25	1920	6		
73	3944	154	886	262	306	370	154	595	59	930	24	1940	6		

Table III c :
Table for calculation of sample sizes
Equivalence of two proportions

P_0 = frequency of the event with control therapy

Δ = limit of difference (the 90% or 95% confidence interval must entirely lie between $+\Delta$ and $-\Delta$)

C_1 is obtained from P_0 (left table) and C_2 from Δ (right table)

The required sample size is $C_1 \times C_2$ for $\beta = 0.10$

For other values of β use correction coefficient (bottom of right table)

				$\beta = 0,10$			
				Confidence Interval			
P_0	C_1	P_0	C_1	90% CI		95% CI	
				Δ	C_2	Δ	C_2
1.00	0.26	51.00	6.50	1.00	10000.00	1.00	08323.0
2.00	0.51	52.00	6.49	2.00	2500.00	2.00	8
3.00	0.76	53.00	6.48	3.00	1111.11	3.00	2080.77
4.00	1.00	54.00	6.46	4.00	625.00	4.00	924.79
5.00	1.24	55.00	6.44	5.00	400.00	5.00	520.19
6.00	1.47	56.00	6.41	6.00	277.78	6.00	332.92
7.00	1.69	57.00	6.37	7.00	204.08	7.00	231;20
8.00	1.91	58.00	6.33	8.00	156.25	8.00	169.86
9.00	2.13	59.00	6.29	9.00	123.46	9.00	130.05
10.00	2.34	60.00	6.24	10.00	100.00	10.00	102.75
11.00	2.55	61.00	6.19	11.00	82.64	11.00	83.23
12.00	2.75	62.00	6.13	12.00	69.44	12.00	68.79
13.00	2.94	63.00	6.06	13.00	59.17	13.00	57.80
14.00	3.13	64.00	5.99	14.00	51.02	14.00	49.25
15.00	3.32	65.00	5.92	15.00	44.44	15.00	42.46
16.00	3.49	66.00	5.83	16.00	39.06	16.00	36.99
17.00	3.67	67.00	5.75	17.00	34.60	17.00	32.51
18.00	3.84	68.00	5.66	18.00	30.86	18.00	28.80
19.00	4.00	69.00	5.56	19.00	27.70	19.00	25.69
20.00	4.16	70.00	5.46	20.00	25.00	20.00	23.06
21.00	4.31	71.00	5.35	21.00	22.68	21.00	20.81
22.00	4.46	72.00	5.24	22.00	20.66	22.00	18.87
23.00	4.60	73.00	5.12	23.00	18.90	23.00	17.20
24.00	4.74	74.00	5.00	24.00	17.36	24.00	15.73
25.00	4.88	75.00	4.88	25.00	16.00	25.00	14.45
26.00	5.00	76.00	4.74	26.00	14.79	26.00	13.32
27.00	5.12	77.00	4.60	27.00	13.72	27.00	12.31
28.00	5.24	78.00	4.46	28.00	12.76	28.00	11.42
29.00	5.35	79.00	4.31	29.00	11.89	29.00	10.62
30.00	5.46	80.00	4.16	30.00	11.11	30.00	9.90
31.00	5.56	81.00	4.00	31.00	10.41	31.00	9.25
32.00	5.66	82.00	3.84	32.00	9.77	32.00	8.66
33.00	5.75	83.00	3.67	33.00	9.18	33.00	8.13
34.00	5.83	84.00	3.49	34.00	8.65	34.00	7.64
35.00	5.92	85.00	3.32	35.00	8.16	35.00	7.20
36.00	5.99	86.00	3.13	36.00	7.72	36.00	6.79
37.00	6.06	87.00	2.94	37.00	7.30	37.00	6.42
38.00	6.13	88.00	2.75	38.00	6.93	38.00	6.08
39.00	6.19	89.00	2.55	39.00	6.57	39.00	5.76
40.00	6.24	90.00	2.34	40.00	6.25	40.00	5.47
41.00	6.29	91.00	2.13	41.00	5.95	41.00	5.20
42.00	6.33	92.00	1.91	42.00	5.67	42.00	4.95
43.00	6.37	93.00	1.69	43.00	5.41	43.00	4.72
44.00	6.41	94.00	1.47	44.00	5.17	44.00	4.50
45.00	6.44	95.00	1.24	45.00	4.94	45.00	4.30
46.00	6.46	96.00	1.00	46.00	4.73	46.00	4.11
47.00	6.48	97.00	0.76	47.00	4.53	47.00	3.93
48.00	6.49	98.00	0.51	48.00	4.34	48.00	3.77
49.00	6.50	99.00	0.21	49.00	4.16	49.00	3.61
50.00	6.50			50.00	4.00	50.00	3.47
							3.33

CI_{90} $(\beta = 0.10)$: $N = 2 \times 10.82 \times PQ/\Delta^2$
CI_{95} $(\beta = 0.10)$: $N = 2 \times 13 \times PQ/\Delta^2$

$\beta = 0.05$ (x1.2)	$\beta = 0.05$ (x1.18)
$\beta = 0.20$ (x0.8)	$\beta = 0.20$ (x0.81)
$\beta = 0.30$ (x0.67)	$\beta = 0.30$ (x0.69)

These approximate numbers must be rounded off to the next highest digit

4. SPECIAL CASES

4.1. Equal or unequal number of subjects?

For a given total number of subjects, a statistical test is the most powerful if the numbers of cases in each group are equal. If for any reason the numbers of subjects must be unequal, (for example, unbalanced in favor of the active drug to the detriment of the placebo in order to supplement safety data on a new drug), for comparison of two treatments (13), a power equal to that of two samples of n individuals will be obtained, if the numbers of subjects N_A and N_B are such that:

$$\frac{1}{N_A} + \frac{1}{N_B} = \frac{2}{N}$$

This formula is approximate and valid for the most frequent cases. The increase in the number of subjects that it produces is modest in comparison to the information gained (Table II). On the other hand, when a "single control" (for example, a group receiving a placebo) is compared to several treatments, each administered to N subjects, the efficacy of the test is greatest if the number of subjects in the control group is in a fixed ratio to the number of subjects in each of the other groups (approximately $N \sqrt{k}$ for k treatments) (1,11).

4.2. "Within-patient" trial

In a within-patient trial (cross-over trial in the case of two treatments) the same subject provides results for one, two or more treatments, which substantially reduces the number of subjects required (but increases the observation time for any one participant). In addition, if a subject "resembles" *himself* more than he resembles *the other subjects* included in the trial (as far as the effects of the treatment are concerned), variance will be further reduced, thus decreasing the number of subjects required for ensuring a good chance (1-ß) of detecting a given difference. In this case, the sample size can be reduced by a factor 1-ρ (ρ being the intra-individual correlation coefficient between the results of the same subjects for the different treatments compared) (34).

4.3. Non-parametric tests

It is difficult to formulate an alternative hypothesis for a rank test. If one intends to use this type of method, the simplest solution is to calculate the number of subjects approximately *as if for a parametric test.* We must bear in mind though, that this number will be slightly underestimated if the variables can be considered Gaussian, and that according to how far the distribution differs from the perfect theoretical Gaussian distribution, it will be proportionately false.

4.4. Equivalence trials

To demonstrate true equality between two active treatments, an infinite number of subjects are needed (cf paragraph 4 of chapter 15). In practice, it is sufficient to show equivalence within a margin Δ. The number of subjects necessary must then be sufficient so that with a given probability (95% for example), the given confidence interval (95% for example) lies entirely between the limits of equivalence, plus or minus Δ. This calculation may be made for comparison of percentages (19, 30) or of means (4, 37, 38, 45).

4.5. Intermediate analyses

Should the aim of intermediate analysis be to stop recruitment in the event significant results are obtained, this must be taken into account. The increase in the number of subjects depends on the type and number of intermediate analyses (cf paragraph 2 of chapter 16).

On the other hand, if the objective is to stop the trial in the event results are so unfavorable that the subsequent development of a favorable significant difference becomes very improbable, the probability of detecting a difference decreases little and the intermediate analysis can be neglected in calculating the number of subjects necessary.

Lastly, if the objective is to obtain an estimate of the variance with no rules regarding stopping, the intermediate analysis may lead to an increase in the number of subjects but forbids its decrease.

5. SAMPLE SIZE AND INTERPRETATION OF RESULTS

"Was the sample size sufficient to reach a conclusion?" There are several aspects of this question that need to be examined (41):

• If a null hypothesis test shows a *significant* difference between the results, there is no need to question the way in which the sample size was determined, since *it did prove sufficient to reject the null hypothesis* and the results therefore are convincing. It should be noted that for an identical efficacy difference, the larger the sample size the more significant the test will be. In a very large trial, if the large sample size calculated in advance has made it possible to obtain a result that "is just enough to be significant", one should not think "we were lucky" but rather "we did good work".

There is one question however, although unrelated to statistics, which must always be asked: is the difference observed clinically *"significant"*? Does it serve a practical purpose? The answer can only be given from a strictly medical point of view.

• If the difference observed is not "statistically significant", the conclusion that can be drawn *depends on the number of cases.*

- If the sample size is large enough, the risk of a type 2 error is low and we can therefore conclude that the test is *sufficiently sensitive*. Consequently, the treatments can be considered to be equivalent (but not equal since only *equivalence* "within a margin" can be accepted).

It is necessary to calculate *a posteriori* either the "power" of the test (5, 6, 29, 33, 43) or the probability of the results under a specified alternative hypothesis (12, 13) or the limits of the confidence interval (41). If the difference observed is small and if there are enough cases, this makes it possible to conclude that the hypothesis of real major difference (whose magnitude Δ is determined) is unlikely: this is a situation of equivalence within Δ.

If the confidence interval only overlaps one of the $+\Delta$ or $-\Delta$ limits, it can be concluded that there is no major difference in the opposite direction of results.

- If the sample size is too small, no conclusion whatsoever can be drawn as to the equivalence or the equality of the treatments, although this mistake is often made either explicitly or implicitly. We can only conclude that a difference between the treatments *has not been proved*, although with a larger number of cases, this might have been possible.

Under no circumstance should we be tempted to add extra cases afterwards in the hope of reaching a more convincing degree of significance, unless we are in the context of a sequential method which has not reached the end.

• Lastly, even if the sample size is sufficient to permit a powerful comparison for the main evaluation criterion, it may not be sufficient for other tests designed to ascertain the *comparability* of groups, the *frequency* of adverse events, or *compliance* with treatment, for example. We must be aware that conclusions arising from these comparisons are not of equal value.

References

1 Anonymous. Coronary drug project group. The Coronary drug project. Design, methods and baseline results. Circulation 1973; *47*: supp 1, 1-50.

2 Altaman DG. Statistics and ethics in medical research III. How large a sample ? Br Med J 1980; *281*: 1336-9.

3 Bowman KO. Sample size requirements: continuation. Oak Ridge National Laboratory. US Atomic Energy Commission, 1971.

4 Bristol DR. Sample sizes for constructing confidence intervals and testing hypotheses. Statistics in Medicine 1989; *8*: 803-11.

5 Calimlim JF, Wardell WM, Lasagna L, Gillier AY, Davis HT. Effect of naloxone on the analgesic activity of methadone in a 1: 10 oral combination. Time and cost flirting with the null hypothesis in tests of equivalence. Clin Pharmacol Ther 1974; *15*: 556-64.

6 Chaput de Saintonge DM, Mendalli NR. Power curves in clinical trial reports. Br J Clin Pharmacol 1977; *4*: 656P.

7 Cochran WG, Cox GM. Experimental designs. 2nd edition. New York: John Wiley and Sons, 1957.

8 Day SJ, Graham DF. Sample size and power for comparing two or more treatment groups in clinical trials. Br Med J 1989; *299*: 663-5.

9 Delaunois AL. Biostatistics in pharmacology. Vol II. International encyclopedy of pharmacology and therapeutics, section 7. Oxford: Pergamon Press 1973: 791-2.

10 Derogatis LR, Bonato RR, Yang KC. The power of IMPS in psychiatric drug research. Arch Gen Psychiat 1968; *19*: 689-99.

11 Dunnett CW. A multiple comparison procedure for comparing several treatments with a control. J Amer Statist Assoc 1955; *50*: 1096-121.

12 Dunnett CW, Gent M. Significance testing to establish equivalence between treatments with special reference to data in the form of 2 x 2 tables. Biometrics 1977; *33*: 593-602.

13 Feinstein AR. Clinical biostatistics XXXIV. The other side of "statistical significance", alpha, beta, delta and the calculation of sample size. Clin Pharm Ther 1975; *18*: 491-505.

14 Feldt M, Mahmoud MW. Power function charts for specifying numbers of observations in analyses of variance of fixed effects. Ann Math Stat 1958; *29*: 871-7.

15 Fleiss JL. The design and analysis of clinical experiments. New York: John Wiley and Sons, 1986.

16 Gail M, Gart JJ. The determination of sample sizes for use with the exact conditional test in 2 x 2 comparative trials. Biometrics 1973; *20*: 441-8.

17 Gail M, Williams R, Byar DP, Brown C. How many controls ? J Chron Dis 1976; *29*: 723-31.

18 George SL, Desu MM. Planning the size and duration of a clinical trial studying the time to some critical event. J Chron Dis 1976; *27*: 15-24.

19 Greenland S. On sample-size power calculations for studies using confidence intervals. Amer J Epidemiol 1988; *128*: 231-7.

20 Haseman JK. Exact sample sizes for use with the Fisher-Irwin test for 2 x 2 tables. Biometrics 1978; *34*: 106-9.

21 Hisleur G. Détermination de la taille de l'échantillon dans un test de Student. Rev Statist Appliquée 1969; *XVII*: 69-77.

22 Jones DR. Computer simulation as a tool for clinical trial design. Int J Bio-medical Computing 1979; *10*: 145-50.

23 Kastenbaum MA, Hoel DG, Bowman KO. Sample size requirements: tests of equality of several Gaussian means. Oak Ridge National Laboratory. US Atomic Energy Commission, 1969.

24 Kastenbaum MA, Hoel DG, Bowman KO. Adequate sample sizes for randomized block designs. Oak Ridge National Laboratory. US Atomic Energy Commission, 1970.

25 Kastenbaum MA, Hoel DG, Bowman KO. Sample size requirements: one-way analysis of variance. Biometrika 1970: *57*: 421-30.

26 Kastenbaum MA, Hoel DG, Bowman KO. Sample size requirements: randomized block designs. Biometrika 1970; *57*: 573-7.

27 Lachin JL. Sample size determinations for r x c comparative trials. Biometrics 1977; *33*: 315-24.

28 Lachin JL. Introduction to sample size determination and power analysis for clinical trials. Controlled Clinical Trials 1981; *2*: 93-113.

29 Machin D, Campbell MJ. Statistical tables for the design of clinical trials. Oxford: Blackwell Scientific Publications, 1987.

30 Makuch R, Simon R. Sample size requirements for evaluating a conservative therapy. Cancer Treatment Reports 1978; *62*: 1037-40.

31 Overall JE, Hollister ME, Dalal SN. Psychiatric drug research. Sample size requirements for one vs two raters. Arch Gen Psychiat 1967; *16*: 152-61.

32 Pearson ES, Hartley HO. Charts of the power function for analysis of variance tests, derived from the non central F distribution. Biometrika 1951; *38*: 112-30.

33 Reed JF, Slaichert W. Statistical proof in inconclusive "negative" trials. Arch Intern Med 1981; *141*: 1307-10.

34 Schlesselman JJ. Planning a longitudinal study. 1. Sample size determination. J Chron Dis 1973; *26*: 553-60.

35 Schneiderman MA. The proper size of a clinical trial: "Grandma's Strudel" method. Journal New Drugs 1964; *4*: 3-11.

36 Schoenfeld DA, Richter JR. Nomograms for calculating the number of patients needed for a clinical trial with survival as an endpoint. Biometrics 1982; *38*: 163-70.

37 Schuirman DJ. A comparison of two one-sided tests procedure and the power approach for assessing the equivalence of average bioavailability. J Pharmacokinetics Biopharmaceutics 1987; *15*: 657-80.

38 Schuirman DJ. Design of bioavailability/bioequivalence studies. Drug Information Journal 1990; *24*: 315-23.

39 Shork MA, Remington RD. The determination of sample size in treatment control comparison for chronic disease studies in which drop-out or non-adherence is a problem. J Chron Dis 1967; *20*: 233-9.

40 Shuster JJ. Handbook of sample size guidelines for clinical trials. Boston: CRC Press, 1990.

41 Spriet A, Beiler D. When can non-significantly different treatments be considered as "equivalent"? Br J Clin Pharmacol 1979; *7*: 623-4.

42 Stephen LG, Desu MM. Planning the size and duration of a clinical trial studying the time to some critical event. J Chron Dis 1974; *27*: 15-24.

43 Strickland ID, Chaput de Saintonge DM, Bouton FE, Francis B, Roubikova J, Waters JI. The therapeutic equivalence of oral and intravenous iron in renal dialysis patients. Clin Nephrol 1977; *7*: 55-7.

44 Ury HK, Fleiss JL. On approximate sample sizes for comparing two independent proportions with the use of Yates' correction. Biometrics 1980; *36*: 347-51.

45 Westlake WJ. Bioavailability and bioequivalence of pharmaceutical formulations. In: Peace KE. Biopharmaceutical statistics for drug development. New York: Marcel Dekker 1988; 329-46.

46 Wu M, Fischer M, DeMets D. Sample sizes for long-term medical trial with time-dependent drop-out and event rates. Controlled Clinical Trials 1980; *1*: 109-21.

21 - Prudence and protection of participants

SUMMARY

Human experimentation is acceptable only if rules of prudence and the protection of persons who are subjects in research are adhered to:
- a research program which proceeds by stages without attempting to skip steps to save time,
- precautions on duplicating a trial (necessary confirmation or unnecessary redundancy),
-possibility of stopping a trial which presents a greater risk or proves to be less useful than contemplated.

Every effort must be made to minimize: the risks, discomforts and disadvantages of the treatments compared; the discontinuation of previous treatments, and the investigations called for in the protocol.

Use of a placebo implies that special precautions must be taken (fail-safe treatment, short duration, exclusion of some subjects).

Confidentiality of the data must be respected whilst ensuring the necessary verifications.

Correct use of results obtained is a condition necessary for acceptability of the trial.

Ethical committees are a guarantee against secret, unacceptable trials.

Free and informed consent must be obtained honestly and comprehensively to encourage patients to become partners in the research.

A better informed general public would be very desirable.

A discussion on ethical considerations involved in clinical research must be made with reference to a scale of moral values which cannot claim to be universal, unchangeable or indisputable. Besides, legislation in different countries provides more or less detailed safeguards which comply with international declarations (2, 13).

1. GENERAL RULES OF PRUDENCE

We shall only discuss the general rules regarding prudence and the protection of persons. They are intended to limit the risks, discomfort and deprivation of treatment to levels that are acceptable to our society and to our time, and are not out of proportion to the expected benefits for subjects in such research or for future patients (5, 11).

1.1. The importance of proceeding by stages

One of the surest ways of guaranteeing safety in the trial of a new treatment is to proceed "step by step" and to decide to proceed to the next step only after having examined the results of the previous one.

• A trial should not be undertaken in humans unless it has been preceded by thorough animal experimentation which, although its results cannot be extrapolated directly to humans, nevertheless enables potentially dangerous treatments to be screened out and eliminated.

• The decision to administer a drug to humans for the very first time is a difficult one and should be made by qualified specialists. Except in special circumstances, this can only be done with a maximum of safety by using healthy volunteers, in whom unpredictable adverse effects would be easier to manage. Administration should begin with very small doses not expected to have a pharmacological effect and dosage should then be increased very gradually.

• Long clinical trials with drug administration over a period of several months must be preceded by *sufficiently thorough human experimentation with short-term administration*. Then is raised the problem of managing "withdrawal". The investigator is also confronted with the necessity for a *replacement treatment*, even if the experimental treatment is obviously effective, so as to continue treating patients who participate in short-term trials.

1.2. Duplicating trials

When a comparative trial has clearly demonstrated the superiority of one treatment over another (or others), repeating the trial may raise ethical problems since it may mean administering to some patients a treatment that has already proven "less effective" than another.

Duplicating a trial can only be considered justified if there is reason to question the results of the first trial either on account of suspicion of bias or because of doubt concerning the conduct of the trial.

Moreover, regardless of the quality of the trial, there is always a risk of statistical error and confirmation of results by an independent study is thus justified. In practice, during a program of drug development, trials that are necessarily redundant are often undertaken simultaneously.

Moreover, if the treatment previously shown to be "less effective" has to be prescribed in a duplicate study, the content of the information given to the patient must be considered.

1.3. Discontinuing a trial

A therapeutic trial may have to be discontinued for two totally opposite reasons:

• On one hand, a serious hazard may become apparent and the decision to drop a patient from a study should be possible at any time if it is in his interest. If an unforseen hazard arises, there must be provision for discontinuing a trial, and even all ongoing trials with the offending drug.

• On the other hand, the superiority of the new treatment or test may become so striking that it is considered unethical to deprive any of the patients of its benefits. In fact, a new dilemma that may be insoluble sometimes arises: should the trial be continued if intermediate results *seem* to be more or less in favor of one of the treatments compared, even though such results are insufficient to make valid conclusions? Experience here shows that the decision to discontinue a trial too soon may be regretted...

2. POTENTIAL SOURCES OF HARM TO PATIENTS

2.1. Serious risks

During both the design and carrying out of a clinical trial, it is important to consider all the potential risks for the subjects involved. Some risks are unacceptable, as for example, any serious forseeable risk liable to cause death or permanent disability (except in patients with a fatal illness when the treatment offers sufficient hope of improvement to counterbalance the risk). Sometimes, however, an unforseeable risk becomes apparent once the drug is in use. Such discoveries probably occur less commonly during a clinical trial (3), than during post-marketing use, since the patient is under "close surveillance" at this stage. Even with well-established drugs, unsuspected side-effects are sometimes detected long after the drug has been marketed.

Nevertheless, investigators must make provisions for all possible forms of compensation and to envisage *discontinuation* of a trial (or even of all the trials with a new treatment) should an unacceptable risk come to light.

Finally, it is difficult to make a valid comparison between the risks (partly unknown) of an "experimental" treatment and those associated with a "proven" treatment and to weigh these risks against the therapeutic benefit to the trial participants. Other "benefits" for trial participants include closer follow-up in the experimental setting than in the usual medical setting, and earlier benefit from therapeutic progress. On the other hand, *a real risk cannot be compensated for by minor or hypothetical therapeutic benefit*. These considerations often lead to even stricter selection of subjects by including in the protocol "exclusion criteria for ethical reasons".

2.2. Discomfort

The potential adverse effects of the treatments compared must be taken into consideration. Indeed, a known standard treatment may not present the same disadvantages, and superior therapeutic benefit over the old treatment is not always expected.

Another source of discomfort might stem from the fact that to conduct the trial properly, the number of visits, biological tests and X-rays may be greater than that required for adequate patient care (even if the extra tests and visits cause no more than temporary inconvenience or simply a loss of time). Besides, it is imperative that participation in a trial should not entail any additional cost to the patient.

2.3. Discontinuing previous treatment

If this is the case, and if such withdrawal is potentially prejudicial to the patient, only patients whose previous treatment is deemed inadequate can be included in the trial.

For example, when a crossover design is used, an intermediate withdrawal or "washout" period is often desirable from the standpoint of methodology. If, for whatever reason, the withdrawal phase is *dangerous* or *painful*, it must be abandoned. The design of the trial itself may have to be changed if it is impossible to assess the effect on account of a *carry-over effect* of the previous treatment. In some cases, a crossover design without intermediate withdrawal may be an acceptable compromise, provided that the early results of each phase are ignored and the evaluation of efficacy made long enough after the crossover.

Sudden discontinuation of a treatment before or during a trial should never be contemplated without first giving due consideration to the possible consequences to the participants, in particular in case of a potential rebound effect, and consequently warning the patients of this.

2.4. Placebo

Using a placebo as a single drug treatment is acceptable without restriction if there is no recognized treatment for the disorder considered (which is rarely the case), or if it is a benign disorder (19), or if the duration of treatment is sufficiently short so as not to involve any notable side-effect, or if a fail-safe treatment is provided for.

Moreover, it is necessary to ensure that it does not expose the patients to any risk or painful side-effect: the selection criteria should take this into account. Withdrawal of a treatment known to be effective has to be offset against the possible benefit anticipated from the new treatment for the patients in the trial (including those who receive the placebo).

All these conditions do not rule out using a placebo in phase 4 trials; it once again becomes very useful in the following circumstances :
- if the risk/benefit ratio of the registered drug is modified,
- if the methodology used in previous studies is no longer satisfactory,
- if the results of previous studies are questioned,
- if one wishes to demonstrate a long-term effect (longer than that of phase 3 studies).

3. CONFIDENTIALITY

The possibility of being easily recognized from information contained in the trial records may be prejudicial to some patients. For example, records will contain information on the patient's state of health that he or she may not wish to have disclosed.

Technical staff, who because of the nature of their work (control and quality assurance) have access to documents bearing patients' names must be subject to rules of professional secrecy.

In addition, it may be deemed *necessary* to be able to identify patients who participated in the trial a posteriori in the following situations:

• *if it subsequently becomes clear that additional follow-up of patients is necessary,*

• *if information that was not recorded during the trial subsequently appears to be of the utmost importance,*

• *if the authenticity of the data is questioned and requires verification retrospectively. In this case, confidentiality cannot be used as a pretext for veiling misconduct* (18).

Hence it is acceptable to record the patient's initials rather than his full name on the case report forms. However, the patient's full name and address must remain accessible at the investigator's to trace patients later on, even if it was not planned to do so.

4. JUSTIFICATION FOR TRIAL TECHNIQUES (16)

A number of techniques may be necessary on a methodological basis, but may raise ethical objections. Such techniques include randomization, double-blind designs, use of placebos and standardized treatments (8).

4.1. Randomization

Random assignment of patients in a comparable trial may be viewed as an *irresponsible procedure* quite foreign to the physician's fundamental concern of choosing the best possible treatment for the condition of an individual patient. In fact, trials are set up because, frequently, it is not known which treatment is better. For example, a placebo may be less dangerous than a treatment erroneously assumed to be effective. *Should there be any question as to which drug is best for a given patient, such a patient should not be included in a randomized trial.*

4.2. Double-blind studies

There may be some concern about prescribing a treatment of which the composition and potential effects are unknown to the investigator.

Although the double-blind design is often indispensable, it should not entail additional risk to patients. If this is the case, it is mandatory to use a "single-blind" or "open" (non-blind) design. An "open" study, although less rigorous, does not, as it is sometimes believed, preclude comparison and randomization.

Moreover, if preservation of blindness represents any danger whatsoever for a particular patient, there should be no hesitation in breaking the code for that patient, regardless of the consequences on the subsequent analysis of results. This means anticipating appropriate procedures for emergency decoding of sealed envelopes accessible to the medical and nursing staff, as recommended in the European Good Clinical Practice guidelines. In addition, it is possible to deposit the code in a poison control center and/or with the hospital pharmacist.

4.3. Standardized treatment

First of all, it must be pointed out that uniform treatments is not a mandatory requirement for a well-conducted trial. There is no reason not to test drugs in their *optimum dosage*, particularly by adjusting the dose according to the effects obtained.

The statistical and practical aspects of flexible dose regimens have been considered in previous chapters. But in the absence of ethical objections, "fixed dosage" trials offer some important advantages which, in many cases, are not very different from what is observed in daily medical practice.

Moreover, protocols of therapeutic trials often limit administration of concomitant treatments, which may be interpreted as a limitation. Here too, only non-inclusion of a subject requiring an "unauthorized" concomitant treatment can remove the difficulty, at the price of more difficulty in recruiting subjects for the trial.

4.4. Participation of the medical and nursing staff

If a trial is ethical, it is avowable and there should therefore be no problem in explaining it to the staff, and obtaining the cooperation of those responsible for patient care including those not directly taking part in the protocol. Acquainting the staff with the techniques of clinical trials is desirable beforehand, so that each member of the team understands the need for the methodological constraints that may inconvenience their primary task, namely patient care.

Each member of the team must also be prepared to discuss the trial with the patient, without attempting to break the double-blind code, but questions concerning the treatment and its effects should not be evaded. If the patient perceives that the investigator is uneasy about the study, he may lose confidence, not take the treatment as prescribed or seek treatment elsewhere.

5. RESULTS OF TRIALS

5.1. Quality of data

A clinical trial must absolutely *result in usable information*. It therefore must be conducted by qualified participants both at the investigator's as well as at the sponsor's. In addition, an effective system designed to prevent, detect and correct any errors, oversights or negligence must be set up (17).

5.2. Falsification of data

It should be unthinkable to hide negligence, to dodge embarassing information or to invent phony cases.

Yet, such blatant falsification *has indeed been discovered during inspections and audits, despite the fact that everyone is well aware that such investigations are possible!* (8). Of course, many sponsors and investigators would never resort to this sort of manipulative behavior and it is in their interests for controls to be carried out. It is imperative for any trial liable to result in practical therapeutic applications to be credible. This then is one of the important roles of quality control of data, of the audit, and of inspection.

5.3. Publishing results

Investigators who favor a given treatment may be reluctant to publish their results if these results show that the treatment is inferior to another. Medical journals are also more likely to publish "positive" studies (which show a difference) than "negative" ones. Conversely, consideration must also be given to the consequences of publishing results for which certainty has not been acquired or which might be interpreted in different ways.

Concern for the welfare of future patients should be considered when the decision to publish is taken.

6. ROLE OF THE ETHICS COMMITTEE

Even the most experienced and competent investigator will occasionally be confronted with a serious dilemma (12). Furthermore, he may fail to recognize an ethical objection in what appears to be a perfectly harmless clinical research project. It is for these reasons that submission of all projects to an ethics committee, or institutional review board, is recommended. The specific role of this committee is to examine a protocol to ensure that the interests of the patients have been safeguarded. In many countries, the approval of an ethics committee is *compulsory*. Ethics committees may consist of physicians, pharmacists, jurists, representatives of "consumer" organizations, members of churches, etc.). The composition of the committee will vary depending on the country and the circumstances. In addition, many institutions and pharmaceutical companies have their own permanent institutional review board (1).

The primary role of an ethics committee is to obtain the *approval of a group* for any study in humans, this in itself being a fairly good guarantee against ethically dubious projects, even if two committees may occasionally give different advices on the same protocol (6).

7. FREE AND INFORMED CONSENT

A comparative trial is justified when there is good reason to hesitate between several possible treatments of which the relative advantages and hazards are still poorly established.

The basis of the study, its goals, methodology, risks and the benefits of treatments must be explained to the patients in simple language. It has been observed that if a patient knows that he might receive a placebo, this very fact decreases the efficacy of the active drug (14). But, using this method allows them to choose to participate in the trial of their own free will. Once the trial has been explained to the participants, it is usually not much more difficult to ask them to sign a consent form, not with the aim of divesting them of the right to compensation should an incident occur, but to be able later to prove that the requirement was fulfilled. That patients *forget* this information (4, 7), is no excuse for not giving it to them, but an incentive to improve the informed consent process.

It has been argued that consent is never really totally informed and free (there may be a degree of dependence in the doctor-patient relationship or the patient may feel pressured) (9, 15, 20). It is in fact extremely difficult or even impossible for the physician himself to have an overall view of all the known or suspected advantages and dangers of the treatments compared, let alone to communicate them to the trial participants.

Experience has shown that patients *can be given the option of participating* in a controlled clinical trial, even if it entails some inconvenience or discomfort about which they must be informed, and of course, provided the trial does not expose them to serious risks. Some patients will refuse, but many will accept and will even feel legitimate pride in being part of what they rightfully consider as a manifestation of human solidarity.

8. INFORMING THE GENERAL PUBLIC

In the eyes of the public, the notion of "experimentation" often arouses fear of being a guinea-pig and of suffering from some prejudicial effects. To assuage this apprehension and to motivate patients to be volunteers in studies, informing the general public is necessary. In addition, such information and formation of an opinion by the public is surely a guarantee against abuses of some unacceptable trials (10). This would make clinical research less mysterious and thus less likely to be feared, and would enable prevention of scandals that have a disastrous effect on directly useful trials, and, ultimately, for the patients themselves.

Much remains to be developed and done in this vital area.

References

1 Anonymous. Department of Health, Education and Welfare. Food and Drug Administration. Standards for institutional review boards for clinical investigations. Proposed establishment of regulation. US Federal Register Aug 8, 1978, *part IV*, 35186-208.

2 Anonymous. Organisation Mondiale de la Santé. Recherche biomédicale: code d'éthique révisé. Chronique OMS 1976; *30*: 405-7.

3 Cardon PV, Dommel FW, Trumble RR. Injuries to research subjects. New Engl J Med 1975; *295*: 650-4.

4 Cassileth BR, Zupkis RV, Sutton-Smith K, March V. Informed consent. Why are its goals imperfectly realized ? New Engl J Med 1980; *302*: 896-900.

5 De Wet BS. Medical ethics and clinical therapeutic trials. South African Med Journal 1975; *49*: 1849-50.

6 Goldman J, Katz M. Inconsistency and institutional review boards. JAMA 1982; *248*: 197-202.

7 Hassar M, Weintraub M. "Uninformed" consent and the healthy volunteer: an analysis of patient volunteers in a clinical trial of a new anti-inflammatory drug. Clin Pharmacol Ther 1975; *20*: 379-84.

8 Kelsey FO. Biomedical monitoring. J Clin Pharmacol 1978; *18*: 3-9.

9 Laforet EG. The fiction of informed consent. J Amer Med Assoc 1976; *235*: 1579-85.

10 Pappworth MH. Human guinea-pig. Harmondsworth: Penguin books, 1969.

11 Passamani E. Clinical trials: are they ethical ? New Engl J Med 1991; *324*: 1589-92.

12 Rosenheim ML. Supervision of the ethics of clinical investigations in institutions. Br Med J 1967; *3*: 429-30.

13 Rouzioux JM. Codes éthiques et essais thérapeutiques. Méd Hyg 1981; *39*: 2616-8.

14 Skovlund E. Should we tell trial patients that they might receive placebo ? Lancet 1991; *33*: 1041.

15 Spiro HM. Constraint and consent on being a patient and a subject. New Engl J Med 1975; *293*: 1134-5.

16 Spriet A. Ethique et méthodologie. J Pharm Clin 1988; *hors série n° II*: 3-13.

17 Spriet A, Dupin-Spriet T. a) Bonne pratique des essais cliniques des médicaments. Bâle: Karger, 1990. b) Good practice of clinical drug trials. Basel: Karger, 1992.

18 Sullivan FW. Peer review and professional ethics. Amer J Psychiatry 1977; *134*: 186-8.

19 Vrhovac B. Placebo and its importance in medicine. Int J Clin Pharmacol 1977; *15*: 161-5.

20 Whalan DJ. The ethics and morality of clinical trials in man. Med J Australia 1975; *1*: 491-4.

22 - Preparing a protocol

SUMMARY   *A list of approximately 200 questions is proposed which it is desirable to ask before starting a clinical trial.* The systematic verification of items presented should make it possible to avoid *conducting a trial that is not convincing.*

When a clinical trial protocol has been written, even if done very carefully, it is highly likely that one has forgotten something (and occasionally many things). Experience has proven this although one realizes it almost always too late.

This chapter contains a list of questions that we should systematically ask ourselves before starting a clinical trial. All questions are not relevant to all trials. In addition, this list is clearly incomplete.

Other checklists have been published in several forms: as a list of "key words" (1, 5, 7), or a review of some basic principles (6), a systematic review of all the methodology of clinical trials (4), a general protocol schedule (3, 5) or as an aid in assessment for an editorial committee (2).

1. AIM   Is it clearly defined?

What can the results demonstrate compared to present knowledge?

Is it known whether there are any other concomitant trials whose aim is to try to answer the same questions?

Have the following been defined:
- what is the principal objective?
- what are the accessory objectives?

Can the trial provide useful information?

What is the true rationale for this trial?

2. PATIENT SELECTION

Have the precise diagnostic limits of the disease to be treated been defined?

How will "marginal" or "borderline" cases be handled?

Has an operational definition (quantitative if possible) of the limits of severity been provided?

What are the clinical forms of the disease which will be included or excluded from the study (symptomatic, etiologic, the rate and extent of evolution, complications, duration, and risk factors)?

Have the three categories of criteria of exclusion been planned?
- as a precaution against some risks for the patients
- as an impossibility to assess
- as a possibility of lost to follow-up?

For example:
- Age limits (upper, lower),
- Sex,
- Pregnancy,
- Inpatients or outpatients,
- Patients admitted after an initial period of stabilization (the length of the period as well as the number of tests for stability must be defined),
- Associated disorders, e.g. renal insufficiency (defined according to precise criteria),
- Concomitant treatments,
- Contraindications to using one of the study treatments,
- Subjects who are not likely to be followed-up or not comply with treatment (with no permanent home, without any family, with little motivation, or persons opposed to trials).

Has an "entry log-book" been provided for to check a posteriori the characteristics of the excluded patients ?

Is the selection specifically oriented to the formation of groups that are:
- homogeneous?
- representative? (from which category of patients ?)

Is recruitment realistically understood?
- From which data?
- How will it affect the expected duration of the trial?

3. CRITERIA FOR EVALUATION

What are the main criteria upon which the treatments will be compared?

Have multiple criteria been provided? Have "composite index" criteria been set up (validated)?

Are the techniques and conditions for measurement precisely described?

What about the metrological qualities of the evaluation criteria?
- sensitivity,
- specificity,
- reproducibility.

Do these data come from:
- the investigator's own practice?
- the literature?
- a previous trial?

The schedule of tests: is the timing of the checkups clinically relevant in the context of drug intake schedules, disease course, etc. ?

Will assessments be made by:
- a trained rater?
- always the same rater during the whole trial?
- always the same rater for a given patient? (is there an acceptable solution for replacing this rater in the case of absences?)
- by two independent observers?

4. DATA COLLECTION

What information will be used to check the comparability of the groups:
- demographic characteristics,
- physiological characteristics,
- onset of symptoms,
- prognostic factors,
- concomitant therapy?

Results: is there enough room for noting each result?

Is there a logical order in the succession of data collected?
Have the advantages and disadvantages of the order chosen been considered?

Clinical tolerability (safety) (serious adverse events)

Is the questionnaire open, closed or both?
Have questions been asked about:
- severity (or intensity) of adverse effects?
- the measures taken to correct them? (including stopping treatment)
- the outcome of these measures?

Serious adverse events

Has collection of the necessary information been provided for?

Laboratory evaluation

Which tests will be performed?
Will they be required before and after the trial?
Which units are chosen? Methods of measurement?
Justification of the tests required:
- toxicology
- previous experience
- systematically

Compliance

Will compliance be measured?
What are the criteria for determining compliance?
- questionnaire
- tablet count
- marker
- measurement of the drug in biological fluids
- recording device incorporated in the packaging ...

Have memory aids or particular packaging to facilitate compliance with therapy been provided for?

Case report forms

Was it judged to be practical by those who had to fill it out?
Has someone done a trial run?

Will all the collected information be necessary? (corollary: will it all be used?)

Can the necessary information be collected completely?

Quality control of data
Who will be responsible for data quality control?
Who will receive duplicate copies (self-copying)?
How will they circulate?

5. EXPERIMENTAL DESIGN

Will the comparison involve:
- matched subjects (on which criteria?)
- parallel groups
- intraindividual (within-patient)? If so, has a possible carry-over effect been taken into account?
  - crossover
  - latin square (will succession effects be taken into account)
  - incomplete blocks
- Factorial design considering:
  - concomitant treatments
  - prognostic factors
  - external factors

Is there to be a wash-out period? (intermediate wash-out) of sufficient duration? Is it provided for? Is there a risk of a rebound effect?

6. ALLOCATION OF PATIENTS TO TREATMENTS

What sort of randomization is planned?

Will treatment be assigned to each patient:
- by packing number?
- by telephone?
- by remote-data entry?

Is the trial balanced on the basis of prognostic factors?
- stratification (how may strata? Not too many? Are their limits not ambiguous?)
- minimization
- another procedure

According to which prognostic factors?

What is the justification for this? Epidemiological studies? Previous studies? Personal experience?

7. BLINDNESS

Will the trial be performed:
- single-blind? Blind patient or blind observer?
- or in double-blind fashion? Who holds the code?

In an emergency how will the code be broken?

Individual envelopes? Is it possible to "violate" them (steam, transillumination?)

Has the code been given to a poison control center?

Will all the envelopes be checked at the end of the trial?

Reality of the double-blindness

Has a jury been asked to discover dissimilarity (of the product and of the package)?

Can the code be easily broken through the clinical effects (beneficial or adverse)?

8. TREATMENTS

8.1. The treatments to be compared:

Which treatments are to be compared?

Do we compare a new treatment with:
- a placebo (justification)?
- a standard treatment of unarguable proven efficacy?

Are the doses, pharmaceutical formulation and indication chosen registered in the country where the trial is to take place?

Will the dosage be:
- fixed?
- changed according to predetermined steps?
- corrected for weight, body area, and severity of symptoms?
- adjusted according to the clinical results, adverse effects, plasma levels?
- will there be a period of adjustment of dosage?

What is the timing of drug intake?

Are treatments compared to be administered equitably (dose, duration, and time of administration)?

If one of the drugs compared is presented in a new formulation, what about its bioavailability?

Packaging

Are packages numbered for use in sequence?
If applicable, is it written on the package that it must be brought back toge-

ther with any remaining contents at the next visit?

How will shipping, reception and drug dispensation be handled?

Has a therapy been recommended for continuing treatment at the end of a double-blind study?

8.2. Wash-out

Has a wash-out period for previous treatments been provided for?

Is it long enough to assess stability of the disorder under study?

Does the risk of a rebound effect exist?

8.3. Concomitant treatments

During the trial, which associated drugs will be:
- always necessary?
- prescribed rarely or occasionally?
- unauthorized?

Will the results of comparison be assessed through the consumption of another drug?

Will it be important to consider diet, or alcohol consumption?

9. DATA ANALYSIS PLANNED IN THE PROTOCOL

What are the criteria for the comparability of groups?

Which are the hypotheses to be tested?

Will it be a one-tailed comparison? (justification)?

What about the statistical methods to be used?

Have the conditions for applicability been laid out?

What level of significance is required?

Have the following been considered?:
- covariates (e.g. initial level of the judgment criteria)?
- prognostic factors?

On what basis have they been chosen?

Are interim analyses planned?
- Who will decide to undertake them?
- Who will do them?
- With which method?
- Who will know the results?
- can the decision to stop the trial be taken according to the interim data? According to which criteria?

10. NUMBER OF CASES

Was it possible to estimate the sample size? On what basis?

Was patient accrural considered?

Was the recruitment realistically assessed? Is there a quantified estimate?

11. IMPERFECT DATA

Has a checklist for missing data been prepared? (reasons: failure, intolerance, lost to follow-up, lost data)?

Is there a system for reminding patients or investigating losses to follow-up? (telephone, mail, home calls?)

How will the following items be considered in the analysis:
- subjects lost to follow-up?
- withdrawal from therapy?
- missing data?
- protocol violations?

Will the arbitrary decisions be taken "blind" by an independent assessor?

12. PROTECTION OF SUBJECTS

Have the possible objections of an ethics committee been anticipated?

Have the painful or dangerous aspects of the treatment or of the investigations required been considered?

How is the consent planned?

Is the information clear, complete, and comprehensible for a lay person?

13. MULTICENTER TRIALS

Is the number of patients to be recruited in each center estimated? (even approximately)?

Is substitution of a center not up to standard envisaged?

Is there a coordinator: its role in the different steps of the trial?
- preparation?
- conduct?
- analysis and interpretation of results?

Have investigators meetings been planned? Timetable for meetings?

Do the terms used have the same meaning for everyone? (translation?)

Is a pilot trial planned?
- to check centers and their recruitment?
- to check the protocol and data collection forms?
- to obtain data which will permit an estimate of the sample size?

References

1   Anonymous. Clinical trials unit. Department of pharmacology and therapeutics. London hospital. Medical college, London. Aide-memoire for preparing clinical trial protocols. Br Med J 1977; *1*: 1323-4.

2   Gardner MJ, Machin D, Campbell MJ. Use of check-lists in assessing the statistical content of medical studies. Br Med J 1986; *292*: 810-2.

3   Perrier CV, Assai JP, Donath A, Roux JL. Directives pour la rédaction d'un protocole de recherche. Méd Hyg 1975; *33*: 461-2.

4   Ryan JC, Fischer JW. Management of clinical research "architecture". J Clin Pharmacol 1974; *14*: 233-48.

5   Spriet A, Dupin-Spriet T. a) Bonne Pratique des essais cliniques des médicaments. Bâle: Karger, 1990. b) Good practice of clinical drug trials. Basel: Karger, 1992.

6   Warren MD. Aide-memoire for preparing a protocol. Br Med J 1978; *1*: 1195-6.

7   Wulff HR. Checklist for assessment of controlled therapeutic trials. Acta Neurol Scand 1975; *51*: (suppl 60) 79-80.

23 - Index

A

Accessory criterion : 200, 254
Accuracy : 230
Adaptative (allocation procedures) : **61-62**
Additional therapies, additional treatments (add-on trial) : 48
Adjusted dose : **90**
Adverse events : 3, 4, 13, 25, 69, 71, 124, 152, **219-228**, 247
Aide-mémoire : 124, 134
Allocation : **53-64**, 155, 158
Ambulatory (patients) : see Outpatients
Analysis of results: 6, 114-117, 125, 145, **164-211**

B

Bayes : 191, 201, 222
« Before-after » : 42
Bias : 15, **19-20**, 113, 117, 206
Binary (variables) : see Dichotomus (variables)
Bioavailability : 3, 16, 50
Blind (simple, double) : **65-74**, 151, 156, 157, 206, 249
Blind-reading : 70
Breaking code : 69, 188

C

Carry-over : 98, 100
Case report forms : **130-139**
Causal relationship : **221-222**
Clinical forms : 33
Coliection (of data) : 219
Combination (of drugs) : 92, **106**
Combination of independent tests : see Meta-analysis
Comparability (of centers) : 141
Comparability (of treatment groups) : 6, 13, 15, 131, 207, 241

N   Nocebo : 76, 80
Non specific factors : 16, 78
Non-parametric tests : 175, 239
Normal distribution : 171, 173, 195, 215, 231
Nosology : 16, 255

O   Objectivity : 39
One-tailed test : 22, 77, 191, **233-236**
Order effect : 102
Outliers : **153**
Outpatients : 80, 124

P   Packaging of drugs : 94
Paired cases : **105**, 195, 231
Palliative treatment : 38
Parallel groups : 97, 168, 172, 176, 195
Parametric tests : 171
Percentages (comparison of) : 234, 236, 238
Pharmacokinetics : 2, 4, 5, 25
Phases I to IV : **2-3**, 4, 246
Pilot study : 4, 144, 230
Placebo (impure) : **83**
Placebo (sensitivity, resistance) : 79, **82**
Placebo : 4, 56, **76-83** , 248
Pocock and Simon's method : 61
Pooling-studies : see Meta-analysis
Post-stratification : 201
Power (of a test) : 113, 232, 240
Pragmatic trial : **216**
Predictive analysis : **202-206**
Preference (between two periods) : **44-46**, 195
Preventive treatment : 37
Probability : 13, 54
Prognostic factors : 16, 61
Protection of participants : **245-253**
Protocol : 13, 142, 159, 206, **254-263**
Protocol violations : **154-159**
Publication : 251

Q   Qualitatif criterion : 204, 231
Quality control (of data) : 6, 207, 251
Quantitatif criterion : 205
Questionnaires : 133

R   Random number : 54
Random permutation : 55

R   Randomization : **53-57**, 59, 156, 207, 232, 249
Rating scales: 49
Re-examination : **206-209**
Rebound (effect) : 98
Recruitment : 32, 141, 142, 154
Regression towards the mean : **30-31**
Repeatability : 41
Repeated measurements : **42-44**, 168, 176
Replacement (of drop outs) : 116
Representativity : **3, 31**
Reproducibility : 6, 26, 41, 150
Resemblance (of drugs) : 5, 70
Risk (for the patient) : **247-248**
Robustness (of tests) : 171
Rounding off (values) : 39, 207

S   Sample size (unequal) : 56
Sample size : 3, 16, 21, 56, 77, 191, 223, 225, **229-244**
Seasons : 15, 42, **55, 206**
Selection of subjects : **28-36**
Self-rating : **47**, 136
Sensitivity (of a criterion of response) : 6, 41, 230
Sensitivity analysis : 117, 152, **153-162**
Sequential (methods) : 107, 194
Significance (statistical) : 6, **18-21**, 232, 240
Specificity (of a criterion of response) : 6, 41
Spontaneous course : 16
Stability : 41
Standard drug : 76-78, **84-85**
Standard pages : 133, 134
Standardization : 13, 16, 40, 141, 230, 250
Stratification : **57-60**, 172
Sub-groups : 200-202
Subjectiveness : 39
Survival (life-table, method) : 116, **177**, 224, 231
Symptomatic treatment : 38, 92, 207

T   Taves' method : 61
Tendencies (extreme, halo effect, central effect) : 50
Time ("blind") : 70
Time of dosing : **91**
Timing (of measurement) : **42-44**, 157
Titration : 90
Tolerability, biological : 2, 132, 231, 226
Tolerability, clinical : see Adverse events
Tracer : 122
Transformation of variables : 100, 170, 171
Transparency : 149, 189
Treatment : 13, 16, **76-87**, 91, 123, 132, 158, 250
Two-tailed (test) : 77, 168, **234-236**

U   Uncertainty : 54

V   Validation (of a predictive method) : 40, 206
Validity of a rating scale : 49
Variability : 15-16, 29, 98, 230
Variance (analysis of) : 50, 173, 176, 195, 231
Variances (comparison of) : 50
Visual analogue scale : 47
Volunteers (healthy) : 2, 29, 101

W   Wash-out : 82, 92, 246, 248
« Winsorisation » : 153
Withdrawn from therapy : 125, 159
Within-patient (comparison) : 56, **97-105**, 169, 172, 176, 231, 239

Z   Zelen's method : 56